10

N. Rey | darebee.com

First Printing, 2016.

ISBN 13: 978-1-84481-007-9
ISBN 10: 1-84481-007-0

Warning and Disclaimer
Although every precaution has been taken to verify the accuracy of the information contained herein, the author and publisher assume no responsibility for any errors or omissions. No liability is assumed for damage or injury that may result from the use of information contained within.

Fitness is a journey, not a destination.
Darebee, Project

100 workouts

1. Cardio Chair
2. Catch & Release
3. Chair Abs
4. Chair Cycle
5. Ctrl + Alt + Shift
6. Docked
7. Power Hold
8. Rainmaker
9. Seated Boxer
10. Stapler
11. Cardio Mixer
12. Cardio Prime
13. Cardio Prime Advanced
14. Fast & Dangerous
15. Fury Master
16. Hero Maker
17. Power Trim
18. Quick Burn
19. Thunderbolt
20. Upperbody Press
21. Fight Ready
22. Full Body Works
23. Glutes & Quads
24. Hero for Hire
25. Legs & Core
26. Lower Body Works
27. Office Circuit
28. Power Switch
29. Superset
30. The Wall
31. Cardio & Tone
32. Cardio: Check!
33. Cardio Grind
34. Cardio Inc.
35. Cardio Mill
36. Cardio Party
37. Cardio Pump
38. Cardio Sculpt
39. Cardio Stroll
40. Slow Burn
41. Eye Rest
42. Hand Mobility
43. Hand Tendons
44. Lower Back
45. Neck & Shoulders
46. Rotator Cuff
47. Sore Feet
48. Sore Neck
49. Stiff Neck
50. Wrist Pain Relief
51. Abs & Core / Desk
52. Cardio Balance
53. Gravity Hold
54. Gravity Hold II
55. Micro Break
56. Power Squat
57. Refresh!
58. Squat & Co
59. Super Charge
60. Time Out
61. Binary
62. Breathing
63. De-Stress Stretch
64. Yoga Fix
65. Facelift
66. Jump!
67. Office Boxer
68. Pressure Points
69. Tai Chi
70. The Walk
71. Arms & Chest
72. Arms & Shoulders Stretch
73. Back Pain Relief
74. Chest & Lower Back Stretch
75. Full Body Stretch
76. Glutes, Quads, Hamstrings
77. Reset Stretch
78. Shoulder Stretch
79. Sitting Fix
80. Upperbody Stretch
81. Arms 360
82. Biceps & Triceps
83. Boxer Arms
84. Chest & Back
85. Chest & Shoulders
86. Forearms & Triceps
87. Office Push-Ups
88. Office Push-Ups II
89. Shoulder Works
90. Upperbody Mobility
91. Back Fix
92. Back Pain Relief / yoga / chair
93. Back Pain Relief / yoga
94. Balance Yoga
95. Office Warrior
96. Office Yoga
97. Origami Yoga
98. Sun Salutation / chair
99. Twist & Hold
100. Yoga Flow

Introduction

Exercising in office conditions is not only possible, it's a smart thing to do. Apart from the obvious health benefits, active breaks increase cognitive and mental abilities, increase brain functions and improve problem-solving mechanisms - making us not just fitter but more productive and effective at our jobs.

As technology advances, fewer and fewer of us require to be physically active during work or do any kind of manual labour and it is beginning to affect not just our collective health and well-being but also our ability to execute all tasks efficiently. After a while, we are simply unable to give 100%, day after day, year after year - even when we love what we do. Being active is what our bodies and brains both need to function and perform properly. The problem is often missed and ignored, the symptoms worsen over time and our productivity along with our health and mood rapidly decline. The good news is, it is easily fixed.

Modern workplaces already integrate fitness initiatives allowing their workers to take active breaks, attend in-office gyms or participate in other exercise-driven events. It takes smart leadership to recognize the value of workplace fitness - and that's why these places reap the benefits of a healthier workplace, in every respect. An active person has a fresh head, is more in-tune with his or her own body and is at peak-performance throughout the day. And it doesn't take a two-hour gym session daily to achieve that.

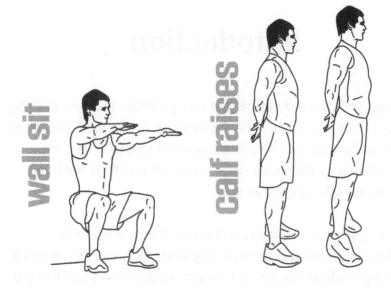

wall sit

calf raises

Even if we only have from two to three minutes here and there to do some kind of exercise - it all adds up. We can all find 60 seconds at the end of every hour. A quick break from writing or reading will not only be a good opportunity to refresh our heads but also the chance to do a quick wall sit or ten calf raises:

Over time, it makes a big difference.

The trick is to find appropriate exercises for the circumstances and the time slot available... which is not as difficult as it sounds. There are infinite combinations of office-friendly moves that do not require a lot of space or even having to wear fitness-friendly clothes. Set a reminder, look for opportunities. Make it a habit.

How to make
the best use of this book

All of the workouts in this book have been organized by category to make the finding of the right workouts faster and easier. Identify the type of activity you can perform and get moving.

Chair Bound Workouts

Chair-bound workouts are exactly what they sound like. These routines were designed specifically to be performed while sitting at your desk. Some of them can be done while reading something off the screen or waiting for things to load or come through.

60 Seconds HIIT

HIIT stands for high intensity interval training which means you work in bursts that raise your heart rate getting your blood pumping faster. There are tremendous health benefits to this kind of training as it pushes you at 100% every single time, there is very little room for cheating. These routines are ideal if you need to loosen up and you are short on time. Another great thing about it is a total time-required control as you can rinse and repeat it several times in a row turning each one into a full-blown workout session. Caution: prolonged high-intensity circuits will also mean sweat.

Lunch Break Workouts

These workouts are meant to be more time consuming and the best way to take advantage of the given routines is to take it slow. The best time to do these workouts is before lunch to encourage digestion. Each one will take you under 15 minutes including rest time allowing plenty of time for food and rest afterwards.

No-Sweat Cardio

Sweat is nothing but our bodies' cooling system that prevents us from overheating. By lowering the intensity of the cardio we still reap the benefits of exercise while keeping sweating under control. It's all about getting things just right.

Soreness & Tensions

Working in front of the screen inevitably leads to sore neck, back and shoulders. To avoid aggravating things further, it's a good idea to take a break every now and then and tend to your body's needs. Pain is a signal that something requires your attention. By not letting these things constantly tag at us we are able to fully concentrate on the work we are doing rather than on our aches and pains.

Step Away (microworkouts)

There are countless opportunities during the day to sneak some exercise in and we must take advantage of them every chance we get: while something is loading, compiling or saving; when we print something out or even when we walk to the other side of the room to make a fresh cup of coffee. The workouts from this section can also be used with a timer. Set a reminder to do one every two hours.

Stress Reduction

We all know that exercise reduces stress. Applied in the right amounts at the right time it can completely change the course of one's day. De-stress using ideas from this section for a more focused and productive, stress-free day.

Upperbody Only

This section focuses specifically on upper body and a no-equipment ways to improve arms, shoulders, back and chest muscle tone - all in office-friendly environment.

Office Yoga

Relax and collect yourself with quick office yoga routines for a better flow to your working day.

Stretching

With these quick and easy stretches you can quickly loosen up and relax your muscles for a total body reset. Pick one today - it will only take a few minutes but the effects will last you all day.

Fitness at work doesn't have to cost anything, it doesn't have to take a lot of time or require a shower afterwards. It is something that can and should be seemingly integrated in everyone's working day - the long term benefits of it are priceless and it is an invaluable investment in oneself and the entire workforce.

An active office is a happy and healthy office that can do and be more.

Cardio Chair

The office chair, one of the most potent symbols of the sedentary lifestyle enforced upon us by modernity, can also become your fitness aid; if you let it. As long as you have two minutes of time and you're not in the middle of a team meeting, this will make you feel invigorated and ready to take on the world.

What to watch: When extending the leg straighten the thigh fully, locking the knee joint and bringing the powerful quadricep muscles in your thigh into play.

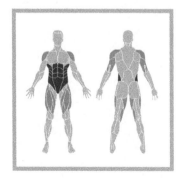

 2 minutes

cardio
chair

DAREBEE
WORKOUT
© darebee.com

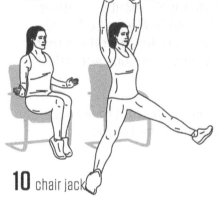

10 chair jack

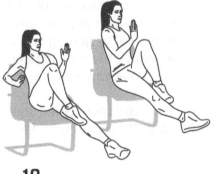

10 cycling crunches

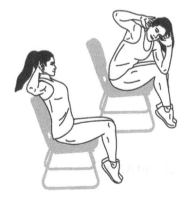

10 knee-to-elbow twists

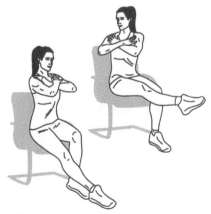

10 leg raises with a twist

2 | Catch & Release

What if you weren't in the office right now? What if you were at the beach throwing a ball or catching a frisbee? While you may not be able to do much about your office environment you can do a lot about how your body and mind feel by getting into a Catch & Release workout that activates the right upper body muscle groups and helps your mind unwind.

What to watch: When your arms are straight make sure your elbow joint is locked, activating the triceps.

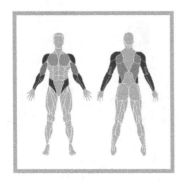

 3 minutes

Catch & Release

DAREBEE WORKOUT
© darebee.com

3

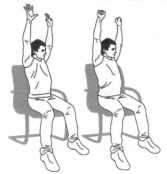 overhead clench **20**

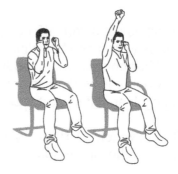 overhead punches **20**

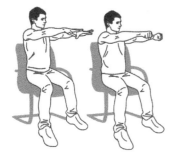 extended clench **20**

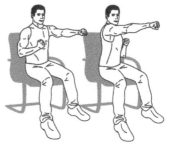 punches **20**

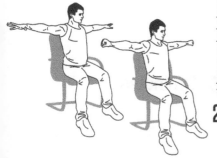 side extended clench **20**

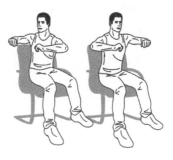 torso twists **20**

3 | Chair Abs

Strong abs and core affect posture, relieve back pain and change your mood by helping release dopamine, the feel-good hormone, in your bloodstream when you exercise. The Chair abs workout is proof that you can hold down an office job and still sport rock-hard abs.

What to watch: Perform each movement slowly, going for a smooth flowing motion.

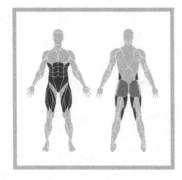

 3 minutes

chair abs

DAREBEE WORKOUT © darebee.com

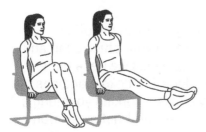

10 crunch kicks

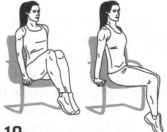

10 side-to-side knee sweeps

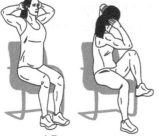

10 knee-to-elbows

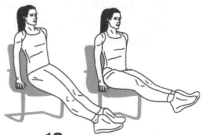

10 leg raises

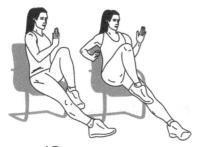

10 cycling crunches

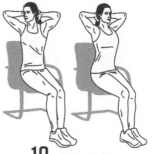

10 sitting twists

Chair Cycle

It's hard to get on your bike when you are in the office working, but it is pretty easy to get on your office chair and pretend it is a bike. From that simple idea we get a three-minute workout that works your legs, hip flexors and abs and energizes your whole body by also working your lungs, plus it's a pretty cool way to de-stress and 'get away' from it all for a few moments.

What to watch: Try and imitate a perfect cycling movement with your feet. Maintain a steady, even temp throughout.

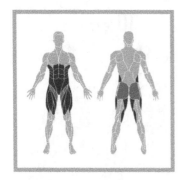

 3 minutes

chair cycle

DAREBEE WORKOUT © **darebee.com**

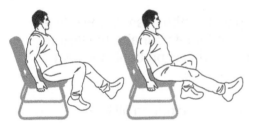

20 cycling

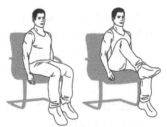

10 knee-ins

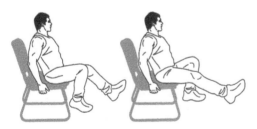

20 cycling

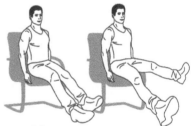

10 leg extensions

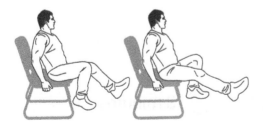

20 cycling

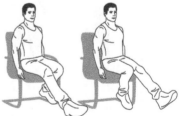

10 slow kicks

Ctrl + Alt + Shift

When it comes to rebooting your enthusiasm at the office a few well-placed routines that target your abs, hip flexors, core and triceps go a long way. This is probably the best three minute investment of your life.

What to watch: Keep your knees straight on all leg-extended poses.

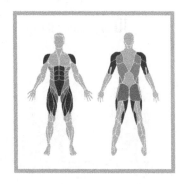

 3 minutes

Ctrl+Alt+Shift

DAREBEE **OFFICE** WORKOUT © **darebee.com**

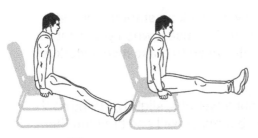

20 leg raises

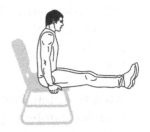

20-count raised leg hold

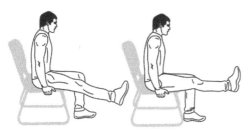

40 leg swings

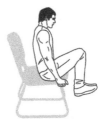

20-count knee raise hold

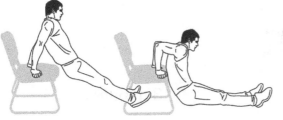

20 tricep dips

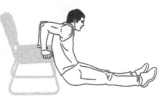

20-count tricep dip hold

6 | Docked

In the office, your chair is your docking station. You get there to complete your work. You use it when you want to get a breather. Now you also need to make it your workout buddy.

What to watch: Pull in your lower abs, slightly, during each exercise, tightening the abdominal wall and bringing them into play.

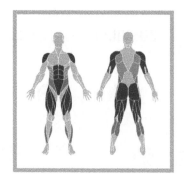

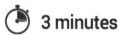 **3 minutes**

DOCKED

DARFBEE **OFFICE** WORKOUT © **darebee.com**

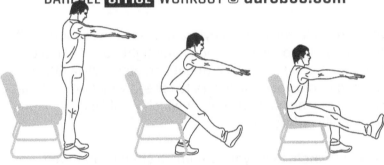

20 chair pistol squats

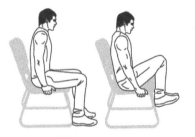

20 knee crunches

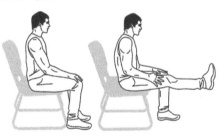

20 leg extensions

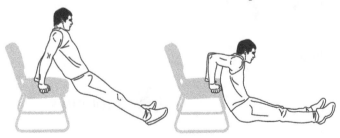

20 chair tricep dips

Power Hold

Just because you're at a keyboard doesn't mean you can't have a totally toned upper body and tight abs. You need two minutes, a little commitment and obviously a little bit of space from your coworkers to extend your limbs a little without risking making contact which would lend your day an entirely different hue.

What to watch: Keep your breathing smooth and even throughout to help your body feel energized afterwards.

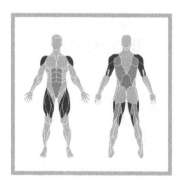

 2 minutes

POWER HOLD WORKOUT
chair edition

by DAREBEE
© darebee.com
hold each one for 60 seconds
8

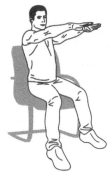

arms extended forward

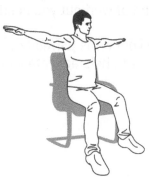

arms extended to sides

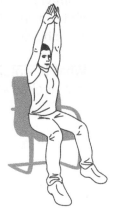

arms extended overhead

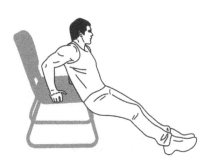

tricep dip hold

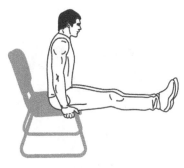

extended raised legs

8 Rainmaker

On those days when you really wish you were out whitewater rafting but have to be in the office working instead, the Rainmaker workout will give your upper body and shoulders the kind of workout you need.

What to watch: Keep your arms perfectly straight, elbow joint locked at all times to help activate your triceps.

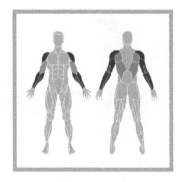

 5 minutes

rainmaker

DAREBEE `OFFICE` WORKOUT © **darebee.com**

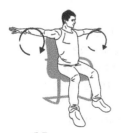

20 side circles

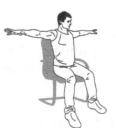

10-count hold

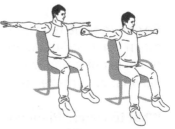

20 side clenches

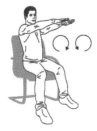

20 forward circles

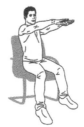

10-count hold

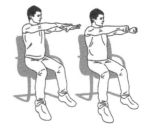

20 forward clenches

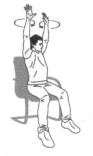

20 overhead circles

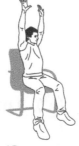

10-count hold

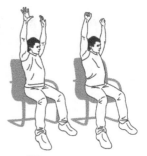

20 overhead clenches

9 | Seated Boxer

Boxing may be renown for its bob & weave but that doesn't mean you need to be bound by tradition. Because the office is not a ring, your office chair will have to be your canvas. Just make sure no coworker is within arm's reach.

What to watch: Plant your feet square on the floor and keep your spine upright.

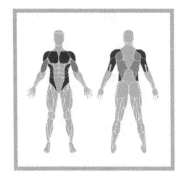

 3 minutes

seated boxer

DAREBEE `OFFICE` WORKOUT © darebee.com

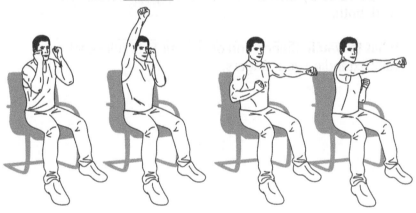

10 overhead punches

10 punches

10 overhead punches

10 punches

10 overhead punches

10 punches

done

10 Stapler

Anything can become an exercise if you do it enough times with sufficient intensity. Fingers are all tendons and they are powered by the forearms. The Stapler exercise will work both.

What to watch: Clench and open your fists fully each time, fully extending your fingers.

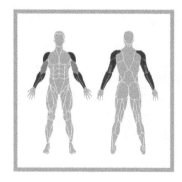

 60 seconds

STAPLER

DAREBEE **OFFICE** WORKOUT © darebee.com

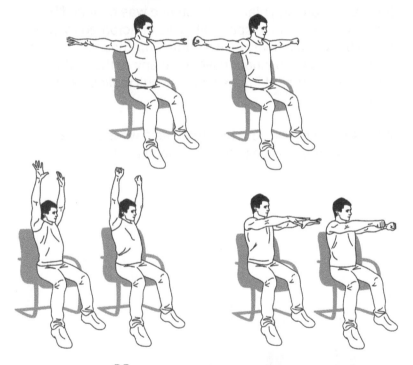

20 arms to the side clench / unclench

20 arms overhead clench / unclench

20 arms to the front clench / unclench

rest & repeat

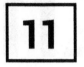 **Cardio Mixer**

Before our roaming plane of existence was bounded by the walls of our office space, life was punctuated by short, sharp bursts of activity as we hunted for food and fought for territory. We no longer have to do any of that but a short, sharp burst of intense activity still makes us feel alive.

What to watch: Use your breathing as a weapon. Breathe out every time muscles contract and in as they relax.

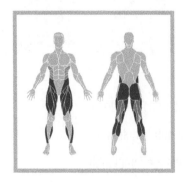

 60 seconds

Cardio Mixer

DAREBEE **HIIT** WORKOUT © darebee.com

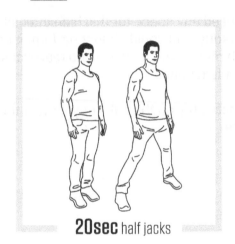

20sec half jacks

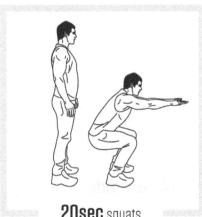

20sec squats

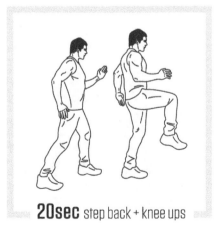

20sec step back + knee ups

12 | Cardio Prime

You barely need any space for this high intensity, interval training workout. You could almost perform it standing in a barrel which means you now have no real excuses for not trying this at least once.

What to watch: Stay on the balls of your feet throughout this exercise.

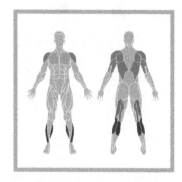

 60 seconds

Cardio Prime

DAREBEE HIIT WORKOUT © darebee.com

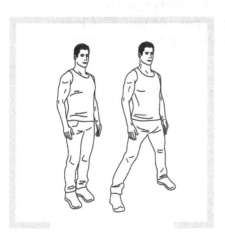 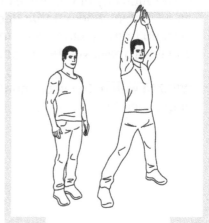

10sec half jacks

10sec jumping jacks

10sec half jacks

10sec jumping jacks

10sec half jacks

10sec jumping jacks

done

13 | Cardio Prime Advanced

On a tough day at the office nothing feels quite as intense as an instant workout that decompresses you. This is one level up from Cardio Prime (no prizes for guessing that) and it will make you feel good.

What to watch: Get your squats to a perfect 90 degree angle each time.

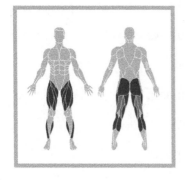

 60 seconds

Cardio Prime

advanced

DAREBEE HIIT WORKOUT © darebee.com

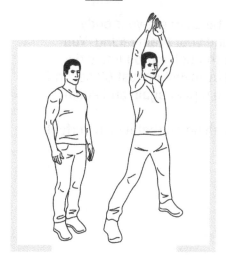
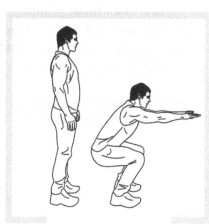

10sec jumping jacks

10sec squats

10sec jumping jacks

10sec squats

10sec jumping jacks

10sec squats

done

14 | Fast & Dangerous

A fast burst of activity is all it takes to get your body moving, your heart pumping and your brain racing. You actually need all of this to get through a productive day and you can gain a real boost by investing just 60 seconds of your time (of course you can repeat again and again).

What to watch: Time your breathing so that it is in perfect keeping with your activity.

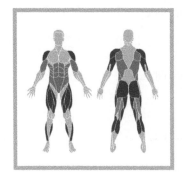

 60 seconds

Fast & Dangerous

DAREBEE HIIT WORKOUT © darebee.com

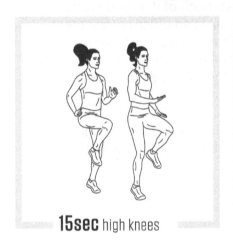

15sec high knees

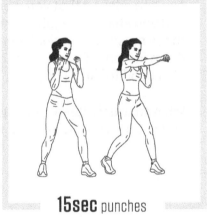

15sec punches

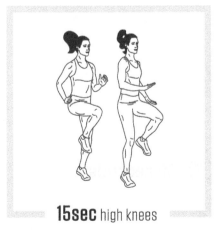

15sec high knees

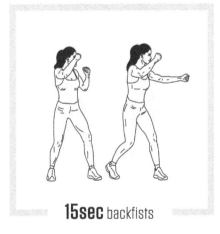

15sec backfists

15 Fury Master

Unleash your inner fury, well as much of it as you safely can considering that you are still in an office environment and you still need a job. This is a perfect way to work all those muscles that don't get to be worked as you're sitting down in front of a screen and the increased circulation is also good for an IQ boost, apparently.

What to watch: Keep your squats to a perfect 90 degree angle. Go as low as you can with your single-leg squats.

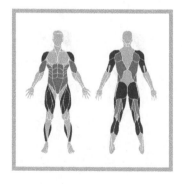

 60 seconds

Fury Master

DAREBEE **HIIT** WORKOUT © darebee.com

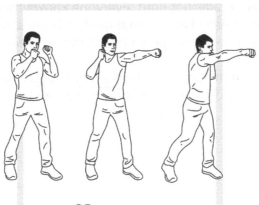

20sec punches

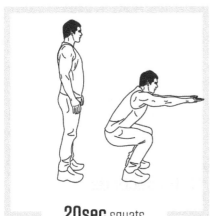

20sec squats

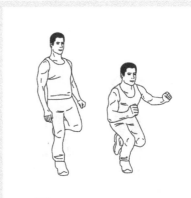

20sec single leg squats
10 seconds per leg

16 | Hero Maker

Heroes are made, not born. Everyone knows that. What everyone doesn't know is that modern heroes are made in the office, in between projects and during breaks.

What to watch: Keep your legs at a 90 degree angle or as close as possible to it during squats and squat hold punches.

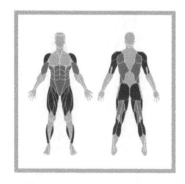

 60 seconds

Hero Maker

DAREBEE `HIIT` WORKOUT © darebee.com

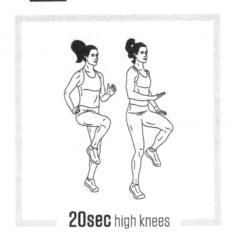

20sec high knees

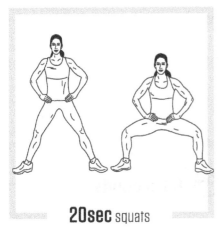

20sec squats

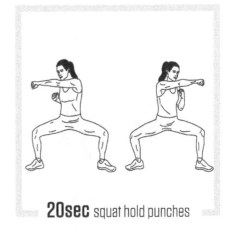

20sec squat hold punches

17 | Power Trim

A trim physique is more a function of cumulative exercise, done regularly than the odd hour spent in the gym sweating heavily and using equipment. Make this part of your day and over the course of a year you will see the results.

What to watch: When doing reverse lunges and squats get your knee down to a perfect 90 degree angle.

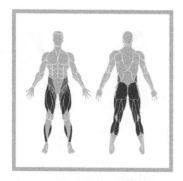

 60 seconds

Power Trim

DAREBEE **HIIT** WORKOUT © **darebee.com**

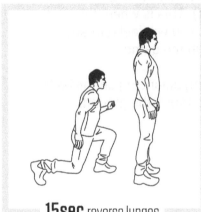

15sec reverse lunges

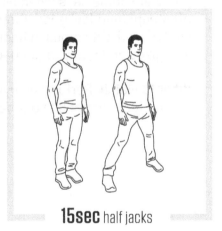

15sec half jacks

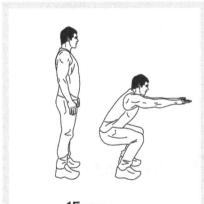

15sec squats

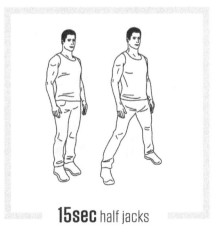

15sec half jacks

18 | Quick Burn

There are some days when all you want is to simply burn off steam (and feel good about it). This is where this kind of workout comes in handy. You will feel refreshed, energized and ready to get back in the game.

What to watch: Perform everything balancing on the balls of your feet. Do not let your heels touch the ground.

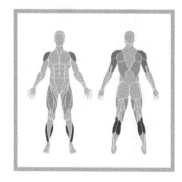

 60 seconds

Quick Burn

DAREBEE `HIIT` WORKOUT © darebee.com

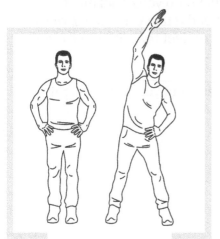 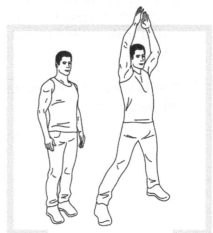

10sec step side jacks

10sec jumping jacks

10sec step side jacks

10sec jumping jacks

10sec step side jacks

10sec jumping jacks

done

19 | Thunderbolt

Even if you were locked in a cupboard you could most probably find a way to keep fit and retain your sanity, which is what makes this workout so perfect for a little "me time" at work.

What to watch: Bring your knees up to your waist height with each step.

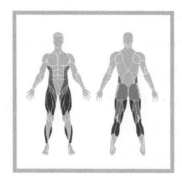

 60 seconds

thunderbolt

DAREBEE **HIIT** WORKOUT © **darebee.com**

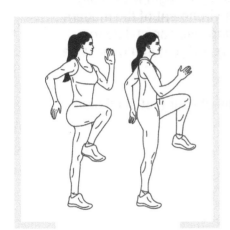 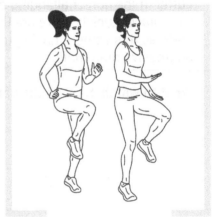

10sec march steps
10sec high knees
10sec march steps
10sec high knees
10sec march steps
10sec high knees

done

20 | Upperbody Press

Our upper bodies, never too strong to begin with, really suffer in the non-challenging environment of the modern workplace. Luckily there are things we can still do to address this without having to resort to hunting massive, aggressive mammals.

What to watch: Stay on the balls of your feet at all times.

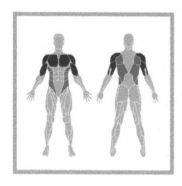

 60 seconds

upperbody
press

DAREBEE **HIIT** WORKOUT © **darebee.com**

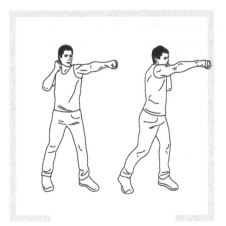
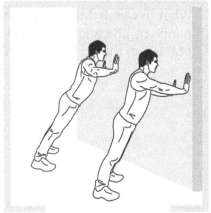

15sec punches (jab + cross)

15sec wall push-ups

15sec punches (jab + cross)

15sec wall push-ups

done

21 | Fight Ready

Obviously every office is a fight-free zone but that doesn't mean you can't use some fight-prep moves to make sure your health and productivity don't suffer because of the office sedentary lifestyle.

What to watch: Move your whole bodyweight behind each punch by pivoting on the ball of the foot that is on the side of the arm that is throwing the punch.

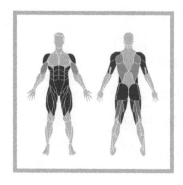

 20 minutes

fight ready

DAREBEE
WORKOUT 22
© darebee.com
repeat 5 times
1 minute rest in between

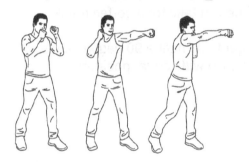 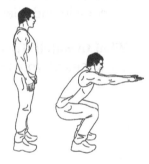

40 punches (jab + cross)   **20** squats

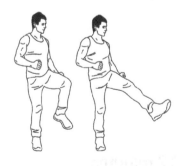 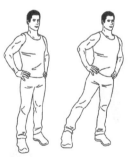 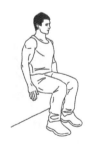

20 low front kicks   **40** side leg raises   **40sec** wall-sit

22 | Full Body Works

Nothing quite works the entire body as this quick workout does. It pushes all the right buttons, activates all the right muscles, has all the right effects in the end and it can still be done in under less time you take for a coffee break.

What to watch: Try and get to as near a 90 degree angle at the knees as you can when in wide squat position.

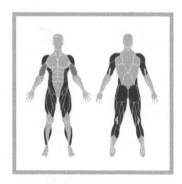

 12 minutes

Full Body Works

DAREBEE WORKOUT
© darebee.com
repeat 3 times | 1 minute rest

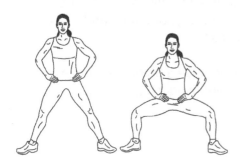

20 wide squats

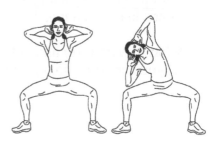

20 wide squat side bends

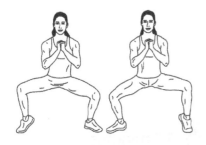

20 wide squat calf raises

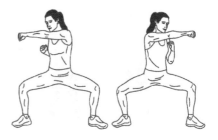

20 wide squat punches

23 | Glutes & Quads

Glutes and quads power our every move. From running across the open steppes in search of prey to climbing over rocks and up trees to escape predators. Admittedly the office environment is a little sparse in prey and predators but that doesn't mean you can't keep your glutes and quads in good shape. Just in case.

What to watch: Try and get to as close a 90 degree angle as you can when doing squats and single leg squats.

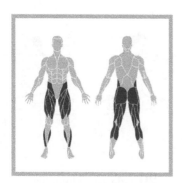

 12 minutes

Glutes & Quads

DAREBEE WORKOUT © **darebee.com**
repeat 3 times with 1 minute rest in between

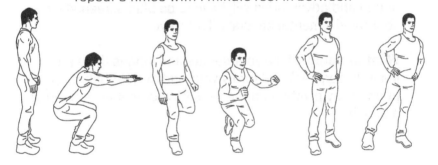

20 squats
1 single leg squat (left)
20 side leg raises (5/5)
1 single leg squat (right)
20 squats
1 single leg squat (left)
20 side leg raises (10/10)
1 single leg squat (right)
done

24 | Hero for Hire

If you really want to know what Clark Kent feels like when he flies off to save the world in his lunch break then the Hero for Hire workout is your chance. You have three sets to complete, fifteen minutes of work in total. The setting, action and adversaries will have to be blue-screened by your mind's mental special effects, eye.

What to watch: Make your squats and lunges deep (at least 90 degrees) and throw your bodyweight behind your punches by pivoting on the balls of your feet as you throw a punch.

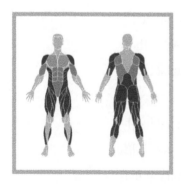

 15 minutes

HERO
for hire

DAREBEE
OFFICE WORKOUT
© darebee.com
3 sets | 1 minute rest

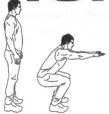

10 squats

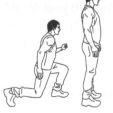

10 reverse lunges

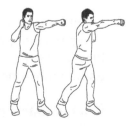

20 punches

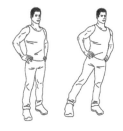

10 side leg raises

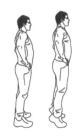

10 calf raises

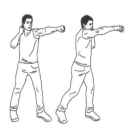

20 punches

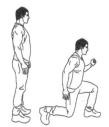

10 forward lunges

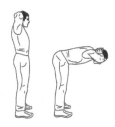

10 forward bends

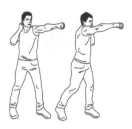

20 punches

25 | Legs & Core

Lunch breaks are not times to just feed the body, they are times to also rejuvenate it with a workout designed to help blow away the cobwebs and make you feel like you've earned that lunch.

What to watch: Keep a perfect 90 degree angle on your wall-sit.

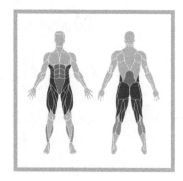

 12 minutes

Legs & Core

DAREBEE WORKOUT 26
© darebee.com
repeat 3 times
1 minute rest in between

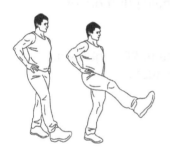

20 forward leg swings

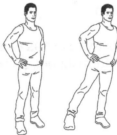

20 side leg swings

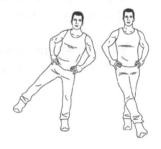

20 cross leg swings

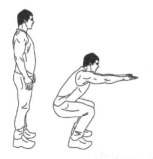

20 squats

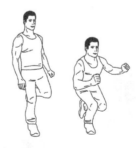

20 single leg squats

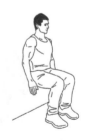

20sec wall-sit

26 | Lower Body Works

Turn a sedentary lifestyle on its head by using your lunch break to work on transforming the power of your lower body with some very precise exercises. These will not only improve your posture but they will also help put more of a spring in your every step.

What to watch: Always try to get as close to 90 degrees as you can, when you perform lunges and squats.

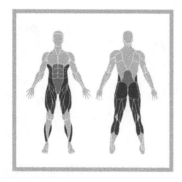

 12 minutes

Lower Body
Works

DAREBEE WORKOUT
© darebee.com
repeat 3 times | 1 minute rest

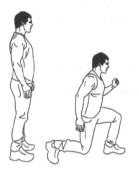

10 forward lunges

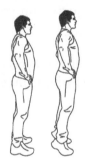

10 calf raises

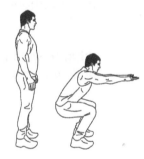

10 squats

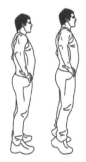

10 calf raises

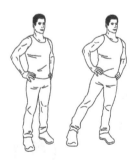

40 side leg raises

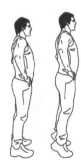

10 calf raises

27 | Office Circuit

With a little ingenuity, an office chair and just the tiniest bit of free space any office can be transformed into a gym during lunch break helping you keep true to your fitness goals without feeling guilty that you're cutting corners at work.

What to watch: Go as high as you can on your calf raises and aim for 90 degrees when you do lunges and squats.

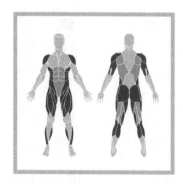

 15 minutes

Office
Circuit

DAREBEE
WORKOUT
© darebee.com
repeat 3 times
1 minute rest in between

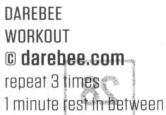
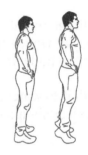

20 squats   **20** reverse lunges   **20** calf raises

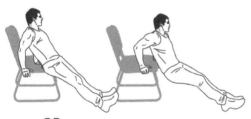
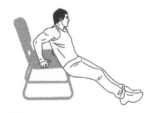

20 tricep dips   **20sec** tricep dip hold

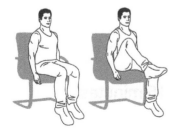
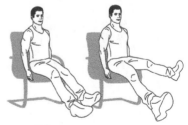

20 knee-in crunches   **20** leg extensions

28 | Power Switch

Fifteen minutes is all that's required to transform a so-so day at work into a feel-good occasion where you work your entire body and, in the process, reboot your mind.

What to watch: Adjust the angle of your body when doing wall push-ups until you find the optimum load for you.

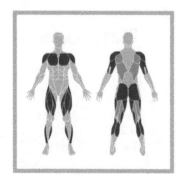

 15 minutes

Power Switch

DAREBEE WORKOUT © darebee.com
repeat 3 times with 1 minute rest in between

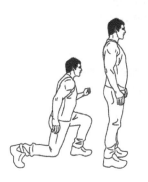
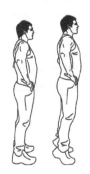
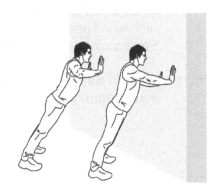

10 reverse lunges
5 calf raises
5 wall push-ups
10 reverse lunges
5 calf raises
5 wall push-ups
10 reverse lunges
5 calf raises
5 wall push-ups
done

29 | Superset

Nothing quite beats a kick-ass, lunch time workout that gets rid of the day's blues and leaves you feeling cleansed, recharged and ready for just about anything (yes, even Powerpoint presentations).

What to watch: Raise your knees waist height each time you perform knee ups or knee-to-elbow exercises.

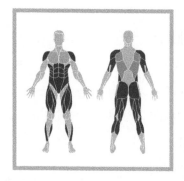

 15 minutes

superset

DAREBEE WORKOUT © darebee.com
repeat 3 times with 1 minute rest in between

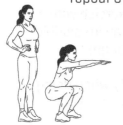

10 squats

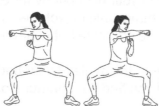

10 squat hold punches

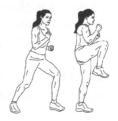

10 step back + knee-ups

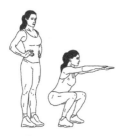

10 squats

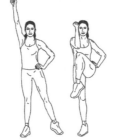

10 knee-to-elbows

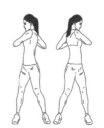

10 torso rotations

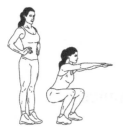

10 squats

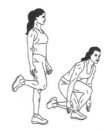

10 single leg squats

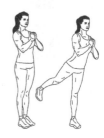

10 back kicks

30 | The Wall

Make your office wall your best buddy for exercise with a workout where an immovable object meets an irresistible force (well, OK maybe not quite but near enough).

What to watch: Adjust the angle of your body when doing wall push-ups until you find the optimum load for you.

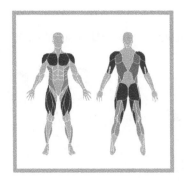

 12 minutes

theWall

DAREBEE WORKOUT © darebee.com
repeat 3 times with 1 minute rest in between

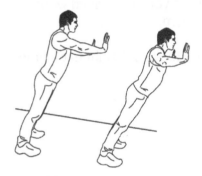

20 wall push-ups

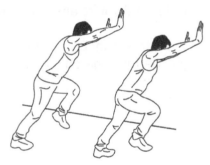

20 wall climbers

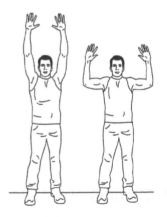

20 wall slides

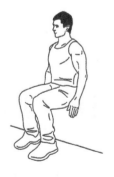

20sec wall-sit

31 | Cardio & Tone

You barely need any space for this office-bound cardio routine that will make you feel like you've escaped work today and you're already at the gym.

What to watch: Bring your knees to waist height each time you perform march steps.

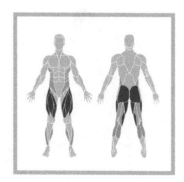

 15 minutes

Cardio & Tone

DAREBEE WORKOUT © darebee.com
repeat 3 times with 2 minutes rest in between

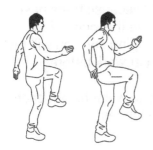

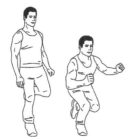

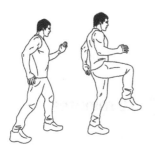

20 march steps

1 single leg squat (right)

20 march steps

1 single leg squat (left)

20 march steps

10 step back & knee up (right)

20 march steps

10 step back & knee up (left)

20 march steps

1 single leg squat (right)

20 march steps

1 single leg squat (left)

done

32 | Cardio: Check!

Office environments are not usually associated with places where one can get fit but that's only because there hasn't quite been an exercise guide quite like this one before. Cardio Check will get your heart pumping and you will feel way more alive than you've ever felt at work before.

What to watch: Bring your knees up to waist height each time you do march steps or reverse lunges.

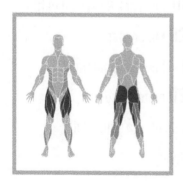

 15 minutes

Cardio: Check!

DAREBEE WORKOUT © darebee.com
repeat 3 times with 2 minutes rest in between

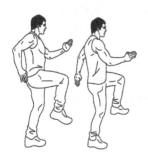 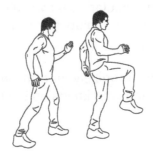 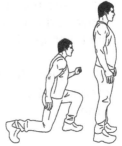

20 march steps
4 step back + step up
4 reverse lunges
20 march steps
4 step back + step up
4 reverse lunges
20 march steps
4 step back + step up
4 reverse lunges
done

33 | Cardio Grind

There are days when you want to learn to take steps in the air and then there are days when all you want is a few exercises, repeated regularly that will allow your body to move and your brain to unplug. Cardio Grind provides just such escape. Enjoy.

What to watch: Synchronize your arms and legs in march steps and try to bring your knees up to waist height each time.

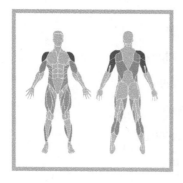

 15 minutes

Cardio Grind

repeat 3 times with 2 minutes rest in between

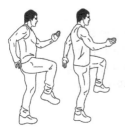

20 march steps

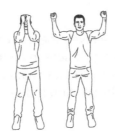

10 elbow clicks

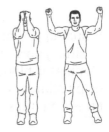

10 step elbow clicks

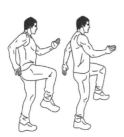

20 march steps

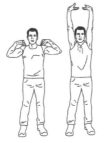

10 shoulder taps

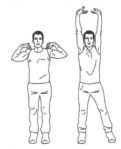

10 step shoulder taps

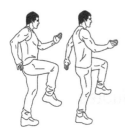

20 march steps

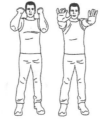

10 bicep extensions

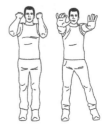

10 step bicep extensions

34 | Cardio Inc.

Standing up not only relieves the body from the stress of sitting down in front of a screen all day but it also stimulates blood flow, oxygenates your entire body and helps stimulate your brain. And it doesn't take longer than fifteen minutes.

What to watch: Stay balanced on the balls of your feet throughout the fifteen minutes of the workout.

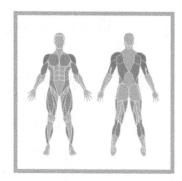

 15 minutes

Cardio Inc.

DAREBEE WORKOUT © **darebee.com**
repeat 3 times with 2 minutes rest in between

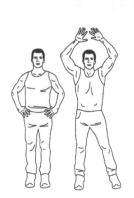 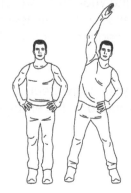 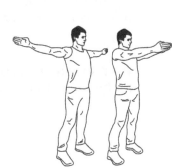

20 step jacks
4 step side jacks
4 chest expansions
20 step jacks
4 step side jacks
4 chest expansions
20 step jacks
4 step side jacks
4 chest expansions
done

35 | Cardio Mill

It's amazing just how much cardiovascular work you can get done my just milling your arms around a little, which is why this office fitness routine will leave you feeling refreshed, re-energized and ready to tackle the rest of the day.

What to watch: Keep your body erect, abs just a little tight for better posture, throughout this entire workout.

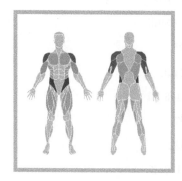

 15 minutes

Cardio Mill

DAREBEE WORKOUT © darebee.com
repeat 3 times with 2 minutes rest in between

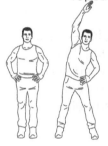

20 side step jacks

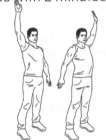

20 alt chest expansions

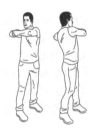

4 clasped arm rotations

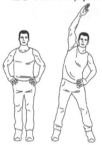

20 side step jacks

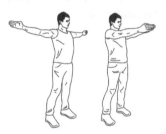

20 chest expansions

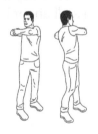

4 clasped arm rotations

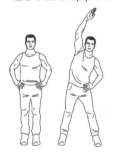

20 side step jacks

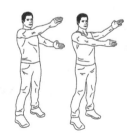

20 arm chops

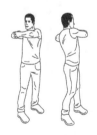

4 clasped arm rotations

36 | Cardio Party

Arms, shoulders, quads, adductors, hip flexors, lower back, the list of muscle groups that are recruited during this seemingly simple workout routine is impressive indeed. If only we could link office productivity to the number of muscles used in the workout we'd be in an entirely different league.

What to watch: Keep your body relaxed and the movements flowing. There is nothing really sharp here so it's all about balance and grace.

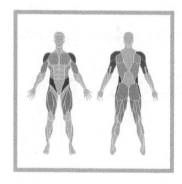

 15 minutes

Cardio Party

DAREBEE WORKOUT © darebee.com

repeat 3 times with 2 minutes rest in between

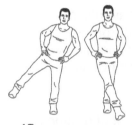

10 cross leg raises

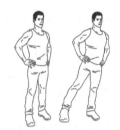

10 side leg raises

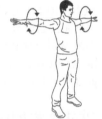

10 raised arm circles

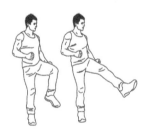

10 low front kicks

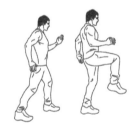

10 step back + knee up

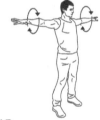

10 raised arm circles

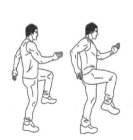

10 march steps

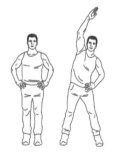

10 side step jacks

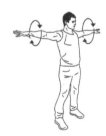

10 raised arm circles

37 | Cardio Pump

Nothing quite changes the mood of a busy day than a quick break for some exercise. This is a set of routines that will get your blood flowing through your body and your heart pumping. The biggest benefit by far however is how you will feel immediately afterwards.

What to watch: This is a fast-paced flowing set of routines so keep your body moving constantly throughout the set.

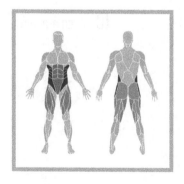

 15 minutes

Cardio Pump

DAREBEE WORKOUT © darebee.com
repeat 3 times with 2 minutes rest in between

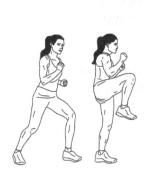 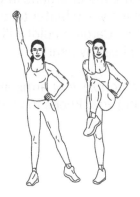 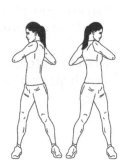

10 step back + knee ups
10 knee-to-elbows
4 torso rotations
10 step back + knee ups
10 knee-to-elbows
4 torso rotations
10 step back + knee ups
10 knee-to-elbows
4 torso rotations
done

38 | Cardio Sculpt

Your heart is one of the major organs in your body that has no backup. That means you'd better take care of it so it can last you a lifetime. Cardio Sculpt will help you in your efforts to maintain a healthy heart.

What to watch: Synchronize your arms and legs during march steps and bring your knees to waist height each time.

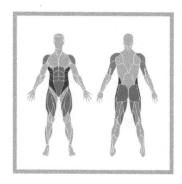

 15 minutes

Cardio Sculpt

DAREBEE WORKOUT © darebee.com
repeat 3 times with 2 minutes rest in between

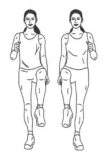

20 march steps

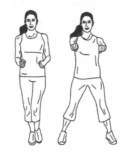

10 double punch step

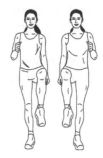

20 march steps

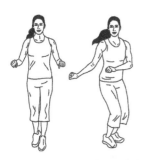

10 twists

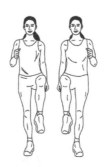

20 march steps

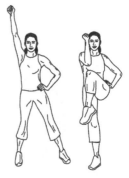

10 knee-to-elbows

39 | Cardio Stroll

You don't really need to work near a running track, a handy hiking trail, a park or a football field in order to go for a stroll. You just need the space you have, less time than it takes to drink a cup of coffee and a little concentration and you've got yourself a cardio workout.

What to watch: Bring your knees up to waist height every time you do march steps.

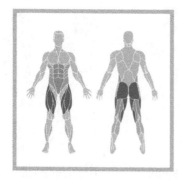

 12 minutes

Cardio Stroll

DAREBEE WORKOUT © **darebee.com**
repeat 3 times with 2 minutes rest in between

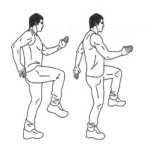

20 march steps

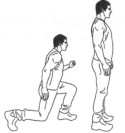

10 reverse lunges

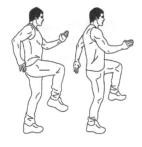

20 march steps

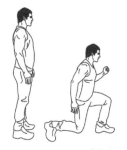

10 forward lunges

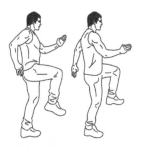

20 march steps

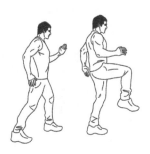

10 step back + step up

40 Slow Burn

Even relatively gentle exercise, done consistently, can produce results. This is an easy, flowing workout that will awaken your body and unfurl your mind.

What to watch: Maintain good balance throughout and, if possible, perform the entire exercise balancing on the balls of your feet.

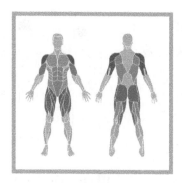

 15 minutes

Slow Burn

DAREBEE WORKOUT © darebee.com
repeat 3 times with 2 minutes rest in between

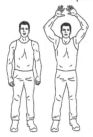

10 arm raises

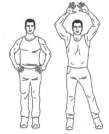

10 step jacks

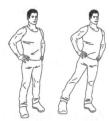

20 side leg raises

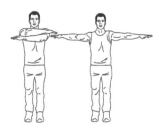

10 chest extensions

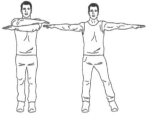

10 step chest extensions

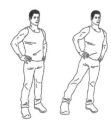

20 side leg raises

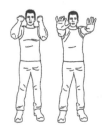

10 bicep extensions

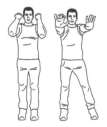

10 step bicep extensions

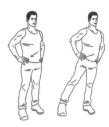

20 side leg raises

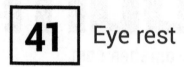 Eye rest

Tired eyes lead to tired minds and tired minds wear out our bodies. Arguably, the eyes are the part we most put to extreme use day-in, day-out, and staring for long hours at a time at a screen, hardly helps. This is a workout for tired eyes.

What to watch: Use the tips of your fingers or your fingernails (if they are not long) to awaken the nerves just under your skin.

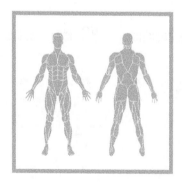

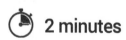 2 minutes

eye rest

DAREBEE WORKOUT © **darebee.com**
20 seconds each exercise.

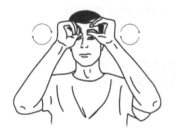

mini circles under brow

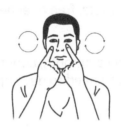

mini circles under eyes

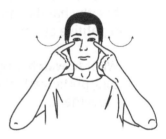

half circles under eyes

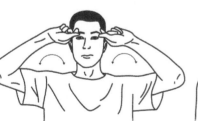

half circles under brow

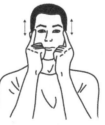

up and down rows
from eyes to brow

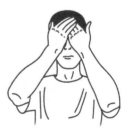

blackout

42 | Hand Mobility

Without our realizing it, our hands take a pounding. Typing, writing, filing and mouse work all lead to a sustained, draining load on a part of our body that is as delicate as it can be robust. Practice this workout often for perfectly healthy hands and wrists, free of aches and pains due to repetitive stress.

What to watch: Apply a smooth, constant motion to this, particularly if you need to develop the full range of movement.

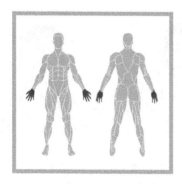

 1 min 20 sec

hand mobility

DAREBEE WORKOUT © darebee.com
20 seconds each exercise.
Repeat every couple of hours.

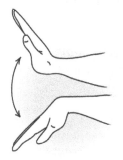

up & down stretch

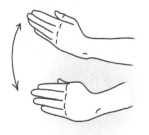

up & down side stretch

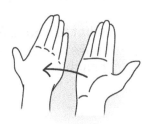

rotations

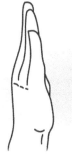 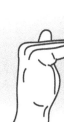 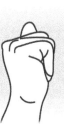 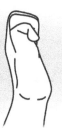 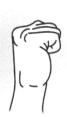

arrow - into - **table top** - into - **straight fist** - into - **claw** - into - **fist**

43 Hand Tendons

The fingers are all tendons so training them to be strong and supple requires constant work. The benefits are fewer injuries, less strain from repetitive work plus supple hands that can be used to do almost anything.

What to watch: Perform the exercises slowly and try and make them part of your weekly routine for optimum hand health.

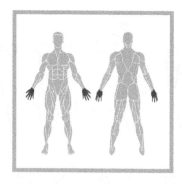

 1 min 40 sec

hand tendons

DAREBEE WORKOUT © **darebee.com**
20 seconds each exercise.
Repeat every couple of hours.

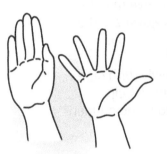

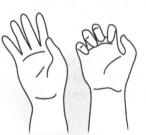

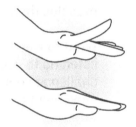

wide spread   claw   finger lifts

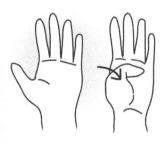

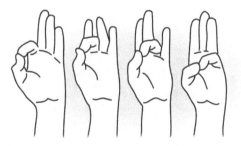

thumb fold   thumb to finger touch

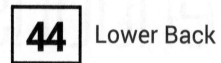 **Lower Back**

We sit down a lot. We walk or run very little. We lift things when we shouldn't. In all of this our back takes a pounding. This lower back workout is designed to relieve the stress placed on the lower back and spine and rejuvenate the muscles there.

What to watch: Perform the exercises slowly, with care, listening to your body as you do. You want to help challenge your lower back and pelvic area so no sudden movements.

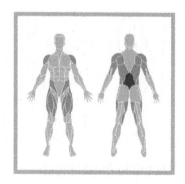

 1 min 40 sec

lower back

DAREBEE WORKOUT © **darebee.com**
20 seconds each exercise.

chair edition

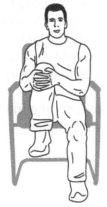

knee in stretch

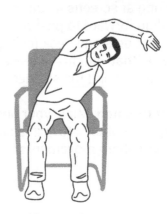

side stretch

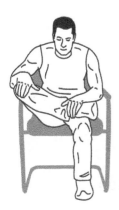

knee fold forward stretch

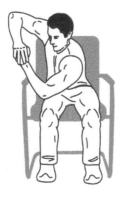

knee-to-elbow stretch

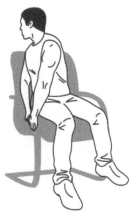

side twist

Neck & Shoulders

Looking at screens all day or hunching over a keyboard or bending forward to peer at our devices, frequently leaves our shouders and neck feeling stiff and tense. The good news is that with just a few exercises all that tension can be released and the stiffness can be made to go away.

What to watch: Move your neck and shoulders the full range of motion. Move in a smooth, flowing motion instead of short sharp movements.

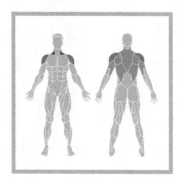

 2 minutes

neck & shoulders

DAREBEE WORKOUT © **darebee.com**
20 seconds each exercise.

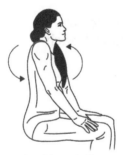

shoulder rotations

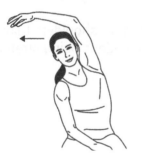

side shoulder stretch

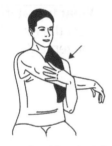

cross shoulder stretch

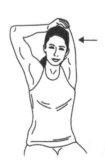

tricep stretch

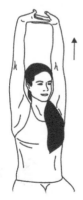

overhead shoulder stretch

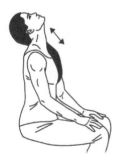

up and down neck stretch

46 | Rotator Cuff

The shoulder joint is one of the most complex joints in the body. The rotator cuff, at the very top of it, frequently feels sore and stiff after hours banging out emails. This is the remedy you have been looking for.

What to watch: Rotate your shoulders fully but slowly. Feel the muscles and tendons being stretched with each movement.

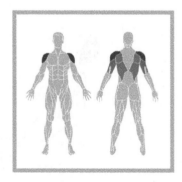

 2 minutes

Rotator **Cuff**

DAREBEE REHAB WORKOUT © **darebee.com**
20 seconds each exercise.

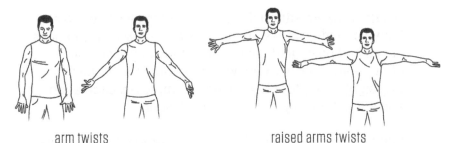

arm twists   raised arms twists

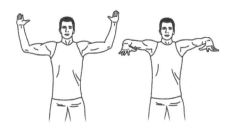   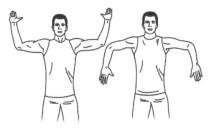

half bow   full bow

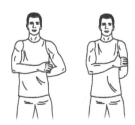   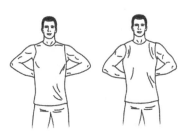

elbow to torso   elbows in

47 Sore Feet

Whether we are sitting down or standing all day our feet take a pounding. They are subject to wear & tear, soreness, aches and pains and get less TLC than any other part of our body. This is where you make amends for this oversight. Good foot health means improved circulation and a great feeling of personal well being.

What to watch: Build up foot mobility gradually. Take care to move your foot through the entire range of motion of each exercise.

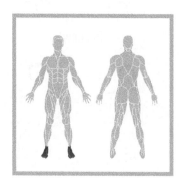

 2 minutes

sore feet

DAREBEE WORKOUT © **darebee.com**
20 seconds each exercise.

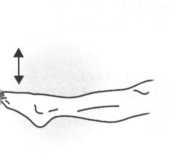

up and down tilts

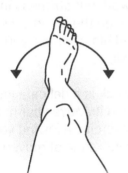

side-to-side tilts

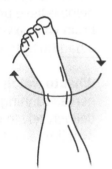

rotations

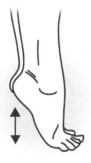

calf raises

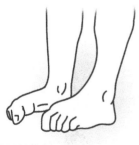

toe curls

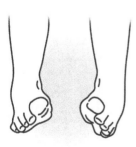

side tilts

48 Sore Neck

Nothing cries out "stressful day at the office" than a sore neck. Being able to work out stiffness in the neck muscles helps relieve pressure on the blood vessels that supply the brain with oxygen and blood which, you must agree, is not a bad thing to do at all.

What to watch: The neck is a delicate joint with lots of nerves running through it. Move your head slowly and deliberately in each exercise allowing your neck to find its own limits in its current range of movement.

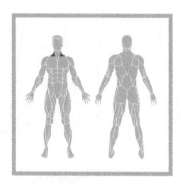

 2 minutes

sore neck

DAREBEE WORKOUT © **darebee.com**
20 seconds each exercise.

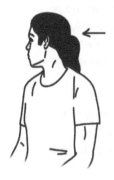

side-to-side turns

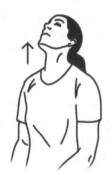

up & down nods

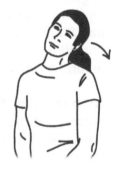

side-to-side tilts

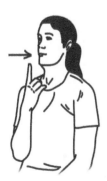

head back

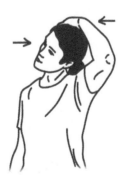

side stretch
(resistance)

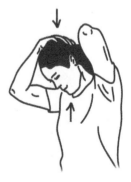

forward stretch
(resistance)

49 | Stiff Neck (Massage)

If you had the kind of day where the pain in your neck began early and it doesn't look like it's going to go away any time soon this workout will transform your working day. Simple exercises designed to help release pressure and lift the weight of the world you've been carrying around on your shoulders.

What to watch: Manipulate the muscles gently but with firmness, using your fingertips. Slowly increase the pressure you apply as the muscles begin to relax, to help you reach deeper in the tissue.

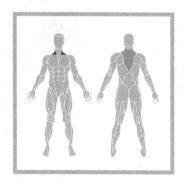

 2 minutes

stiff neck

DAREBEE WORKOUT © **darebee.com**
20 seconds each exercise.

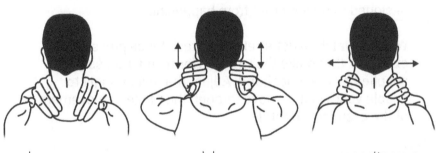

| neck massage | up and down rows | opposite rows |

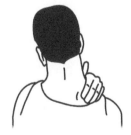
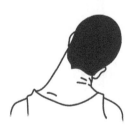

| shoulder massage | grip slides | side-to-side tilts |

50 | Wrist Pain

Repetitive work like typing or mouse clicking is a killer for wrists. It takes remarkably little pressure to inflame the tissue running through the narrow carpal tunnel and compress the nerves in that area. This is a workout designed to prevent that from happening.

What to watch: Wrist stretch and resistance press are exercises that make the wrist perform under pressure supplied by the other hand. Adjust that accordingly to enable your wrist to move through the range of movement of the exercise smoothly.

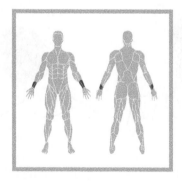

 2 minutes

wrist pain

DAREBEE WORKOUT © **darebee.com**
20 seconds each exercise.
Repeat every couple of hours.

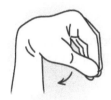

wrist curl

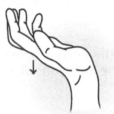

tilt back

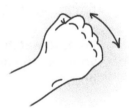

"hammer"

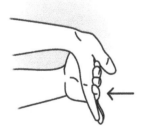

wrist stretch

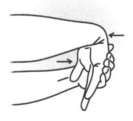

resistance press

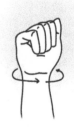

fist rotations

51 | Abs & Core

Desks are not only important pieces of office furniture without which we wouldn't be able to get much work done, they can also be transformed into a handy multi-gym station that allows us to train some of the major muscle groups in our body.

What to watch: The further away from the desk you place your feet the greater the load you will bring to bear on your body.

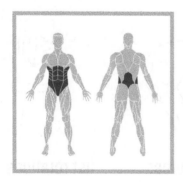

 4 min 30 sec

Abs & Core

desk edition

DAREBEE WORKOUT © darebee.com

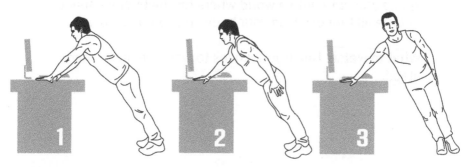

30 seconds
table plank

60 seconds
one arm table plank

60 seconds
side table plank

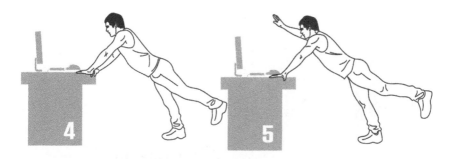

60 seconds
raised leg table plank

60 seconds
alternative arm and leg raise table plank

52 | Cardio Balance

Step away from your desk for a minute (well, two actually), push your office chair well in to give yourself just a little space and enter into a world where for the briefest space of time all that exists is your body and your heartbeat.

What to watch: Raise your knees to waist height in march steps.

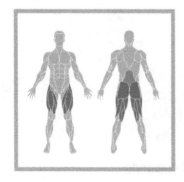

 2 minutes

Cardio
Balance

DAREBEE WORKOUT © darebee.com

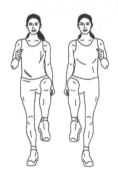 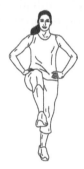 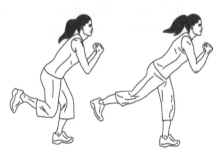

10 march steps

10-count raised knee hold (right leg)

10 single leg back kicks (right leg)

10 march steps

10-count raised knee hold (left leg)

10 single leg back kicks (left left)

done

53 | Gravity Hold

Gravity is always against us except when it is put to work for us and in this workout it is most definitely the latter as we recruit it to act as equipment for us, creating resistance forces we have to work against.

What to watch: Go as low as you possibly can in the single half squat. The ideal is a 90 degree angle and hold it throughout the ten seconds.

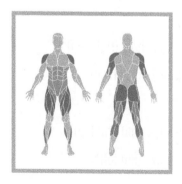

 2 minutes

gravity hold

DAREBEE WORKOUT
© darebee.com
10 seconds hold each.
Change sides & repeat.

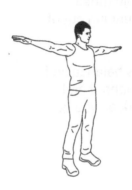

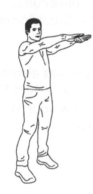

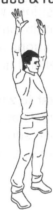

arms extended to sides   arms extended to the front   arms extended overhead

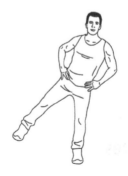

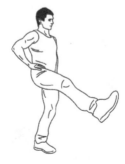

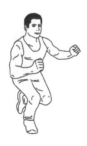

leg raised to the siide   leg raised forward   single leg half squat

Gravity Hold II

Using gravity to help us get fitter requires going into positions where muscle tension is used to help the body remain balanced. The challenge is then to hold those positions against time without the muscles running out of fuel and tiring.

What to watch: The important element here is balance and muscle awareness. Keep a perfect form throughout and make sure you feel the way your muscles work as you go from one pose to the next.

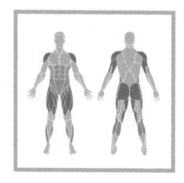

 4 minutes

gravity *hold II*

DAREBEE WORKOUT
© **darebee.com**
20 seconds hold each.
Change sides & repeat.

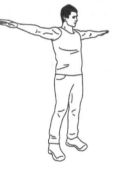

arms raised to the side

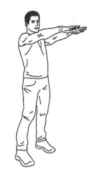

arms raised to the front

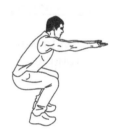

squat hold with arms raised

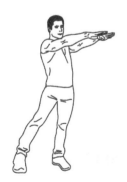

leg raised to the side

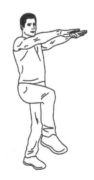

knee raised up

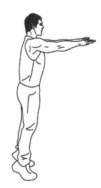

calf raise hold

55 | Micro Break

By pitting one muscle group against another we use our own body's strength to get stronger and feel rejuvenated. The Micro Break workout appears deceptively simple but it will make you feel so alive you'd want to come back to it again and again.

What to watch: Keep your elbows raised to shoulder height throughout.

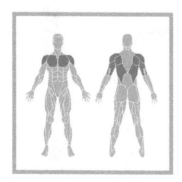

 60 Seconds

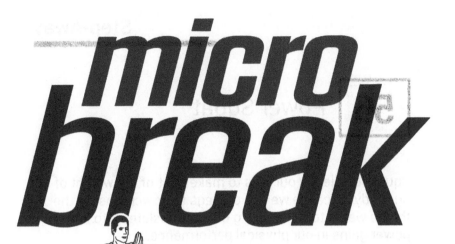

micro break

by DAREBEE © **darebee.com**

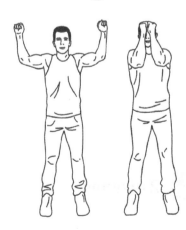

10-count chest squeeze

4 elbow clicks

10-count chest squeeze

4 elbow clicks

10-count chest squeeze

4 elbow clicks

10-count chest squeeze

4 elbow clicks

done

56 | Power Squat

Squats challenge our legs to make light of the weight of our body. Because we use our legs to power most of the things we do to have strong quads translates into real power gains in our physical performance.

What to watch: Achieve as near a 90 degree angle with your squats as you can and rise as high as possible on your calf raises.

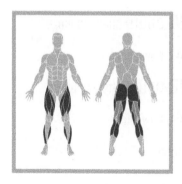

 2 minutes

Power Squat

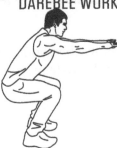

DAREBEE WORKOUT © darebee.com

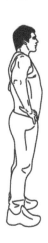
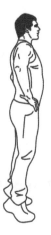

5 squats

5 calf raises

10 squats

10 calf raises

20 squats

20 calf raises

10 squats

10 calf raises

5 squats

5 calf raises

done

57 | Refresh

Few workouts will leave you feeling as refreshed and ready for virtually anything as the Refresh workout. Designed to stimulate your body and mind on a busy working day this should be a natural go-to workout for those days you can spare a couple of minutes and could do with feeling a little well ... refreshed.

What to watch: Breathe in deeply when your arms expand and your chest is thrust out and exhale as you bring your arms together in front of you.

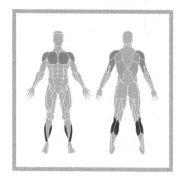

 2 minutes

Refresh

DAREBEE WORKOUT © **darebee.com**

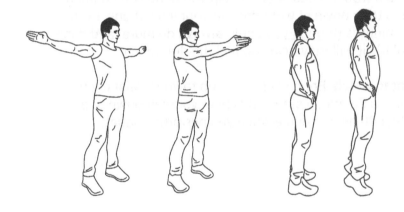

5 chest expansions

5 calf raises

10 chest expansions

10 calf raises

20 chest expansions

20 calf raises

done

58 | Squat & Co

Because we sit down most of the day our legs lose much of their power and strength. Rest easy however because this is a workout designed to help you undo what damage your sitting down at work does to your legs. It only takes two minutes (though you could always do more) and done regularly it will truly help you feel the difference.

What to watch: Bring your knees up to your waist each time you do march steps and lower yourself down to a perfect 90 degree angle when you perform a squat.

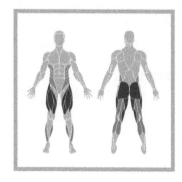

 2 minutes

Squat & Go

DAREBEE WORKOUT © darebee.com

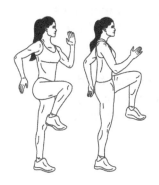
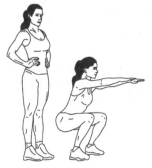
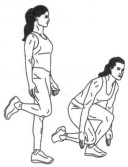

10 march steps

10 squats

2 single leg squats (left leg)

10 march steps

10 squats

2 single leg squats (right leg)

done

59 | Super Charge

It's hard to get a full body workout without ditching work and getting to a gym but the Super Charge workout helps you achieve just that with just a few stationary exercises compiled in a very clever way to help challenge just the right muscle groups.

What to watch: When holding the squat in squat hold punches your thighs should be held at approximately a 45 degree angle, for best strength results in your quad-muscles.

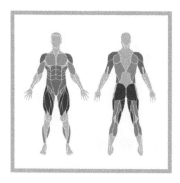

 3 minutes

Super Charge

FULL BODY WORKOUT by © darebee.com

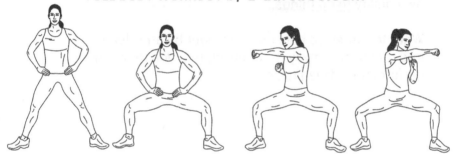

5 squats

10 squat hold punches

10 squats

20 squat hold punches

15 squats

30 squat hold punches

20 squats

40 squat hold punches

done

60 | Time Out

By making it easy to find ways to exercise regularly, every day, you help your body adapt to a more physical lifestyle. It gains strength, endurance and improves its overall cardiovascular health. This gives you confidence in your own ability to do things.

What to watch: To help maintain your balance lean into rather than away from the leg that you raise when performing side leg raises.

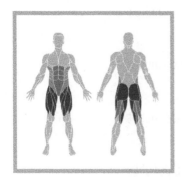

 2 minutes

Time Out

DAREBEE WORKOUT © **darebee.com**

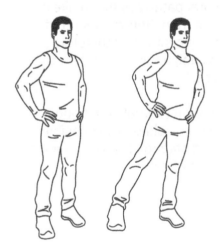 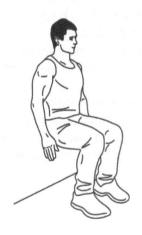

30sec side leg raises (left leg)

30sec wall-sit

30sec side leg raises (right leg)

30sec wall-sit

done

61	Binary

Fitness always begins with the mind. In order for our body to do something our mind must first visualize it and then create the necessary neural pathways that make it possible to happen. This is a coordination workout that truly challenges our ability to concentrate. It therefore goes a long way towards providing a full work out for the brain and relieving office stress.

What to watch: Pay close attention to what your hands are doing. Trace as exact geometric shapes as possible with tour extended finger, taking care to form very precise geometric lines in the air in front of you.

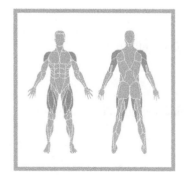

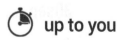 up to you

binary workout

by DAREBEE © darebee.com

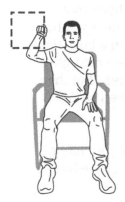

Draw a square with the extended finger of one hand.

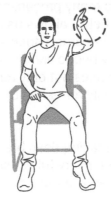

Now draw a circle with the other.

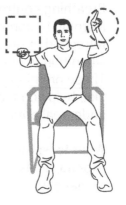

Now do both.

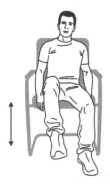

Sitting down raise dominant knee up & down.

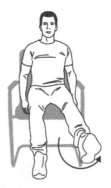

Kick the other leg back & forth.

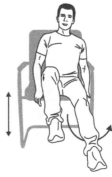

Now do both.

62 | Breathing

Breathing controls so many processes in our body that learning to control it better allows us to determine just how refreshed or tired we become, especially during a busy day when things get really hectic and our chest become tight. These breathing exercises not only release stress but they also help you feel totally refreshed on days when you're under real pressure.

What to watch: When taking deep breaths feel your lungs expand, fill them to their very fullest so that they are forced to make full use of their volume.

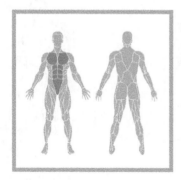

 2 minutes

Breathing
Workout

by DAREBEE © **darebee.com**

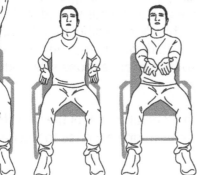

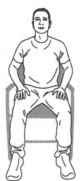

Breathe in slowly, hold to a slow count of ten then exhale slowly. Repeat 3 times.

Take ten rapid breaths. Hold without breathing to the count of twenty.

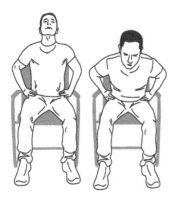

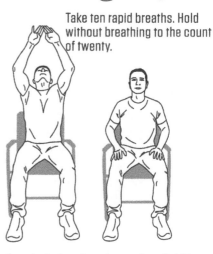

Breathe in and lean back, breathe out and lean forward. Repeat 3 times.

Breathe in fast, breathe out fast. Hold for count of three. Repeat 3 times.

63 | De-Stress Stretching

Stress is a stealthy enemy that creeps up on us and places little knots in the muscles between our shoulder blades, our back and our neck. This de-stressing stretch routine irons all those muscles out, flexing them and moving them in a very specific way to help release those stress knots before they get too tight.

What to watch: You should be able to feel the muscles you are tensing as you move from one exercise to the next.

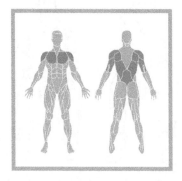

 60 seconds

60-second
de-stress

by DAREBEE © **darebee.com**
Repeat each one for 10 seconds. stretching

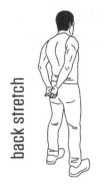

back stretch

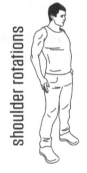

shoulder rotations

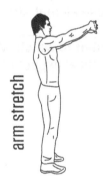

arm stretch

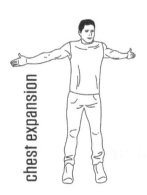

chest expansion

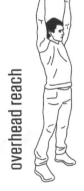

overhead reach

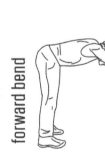

forward bend

64 Yoga Fix

Letting yourself be absorbed by the intricacy of balancing like a Yogi and feeling each breath you take coursing through your body is one of the easiest ways there is to lose all that stress and dive into a self-made oasis.

What to watch: Maintaining your balance is the most critical aspect of each of these exercises.

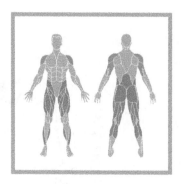

 3 Minutes

DE-STRESS
YOGA FIX

by DAREBEE © darebee.com
Change sides and repeat.

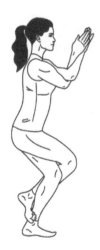
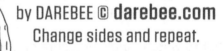
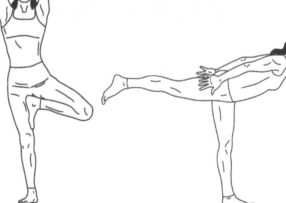

Eagle	Tree Pose	Warrior III
30	**30**	**30**
seconds	seconds	seconds

65 | Facelift

Stress, fatigue, high emotion, drama - all conspire to age us. They tire our facial muscles, drain blood away from our face and add stress lines where none should be. Luckily this workout will help revitalize how your face feels and totally improve your mood.

What to watch: Apply pressure on the skin with your fingertips or, if possible, with the edge of your fingernails in a very firm manner.

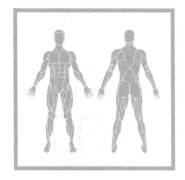

 60 seconds

FACELIFT
WORKOUT

by DAREBEE © darebee.com
Repeat each exercise for **10 seconds**.

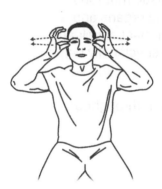

Draw parallel lines above and below your eye with your fingertips or nails.

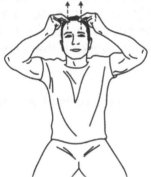

Start from your eyebrows and stretch your forehead towards the hairline.

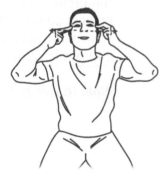

Start from the edge of your eyes and stretch the skin towards your hairline.

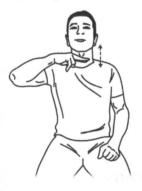

With extended index and trigger fingers together tap rapildy under your chin.

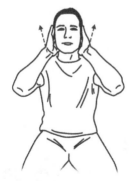

Place thumbs under your jaw and move your hands firmly towards the top of your head

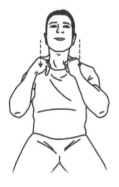

Place your index finger behind your ear and pull firmly to the base of your neck.

66 | Jump!

Fascial fitness refers to the connecting tissue that runs throughout the body, supports muscles and organs and powers some of the body's responses to impact shock and vibration. This is a mini workout that very specifically helps improve its fitness.

What to watch: Stay on the balls of your feet throughout.

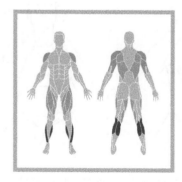

 30 seconds

JUMP!

mini-workout
by DAREBEE © darebee.com

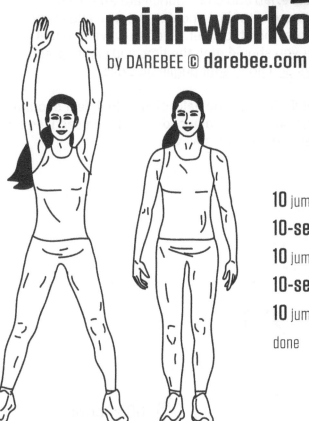

10 jumping jacks
10-seconds rest
10 jumping jacks
10-seconds rest
10 jumping jacks
done

67 | Office Boxer

Bob and weave, jab and cross punch are exercises associated more with time spent at the gym and away from work than the office. Yet, if you truly want to feel like a contender you should grab the time you can to practice some moves and hone your pugilistic skills.

What to watch: Stay on the balls of your feet, feet shoulder-width apart, bodyweight balanced fifty-fifty on each leg and with your left leg forward, always.

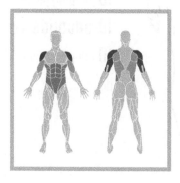

 60 seconds

OFFICE BOXER WORKOUT

by DAREBEE
© darebee.com

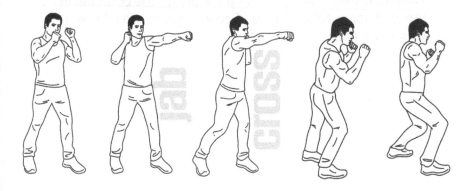

20 jab + cross
2 side-to-side tilts
20 jabs (left arm)
2 side-to-side tilts
20 jabs (right arm)
2 side-to-side tilts
done

Relieve stress
and stay in shape
during office hours!

Repeat every 2hrs
or whenever possible.

68 | Pressure Points

Use pressure point therapy to totally revitalise your body and mind and turn a pressured day at the office into a much more relaxed, controlled affair.

What to watch: Place positive pressure on the point being pressed using either the tip of your finger or the edge of your fingernail.

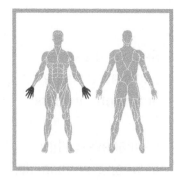

 60 seconds

pressure
points

DAREBEE WORKOUT © **darebee.com**
Repeat each one for 10 seconds.

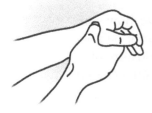

thenar press

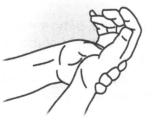

palm rub

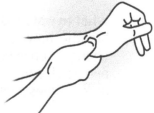

thumb root press

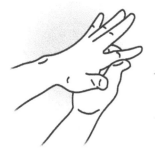

bottom
index finger press

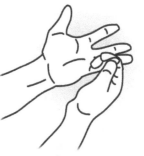

top
little finger press

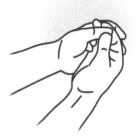

top
thumb press

69 | Tai Chi

Become one with the universe and feel the flow of your life force as you move, body and mind in total harmony, breathing deeply, evenly and in a controlled manner. This one is for those who want to completely recharge themselves.

What to watch: Be mindful of how you move, how you breathe, how your body weight shifts and your balance changes. Lose yourself in the flow of the movement and you'll soon find any kind of self-consciousness and awkwardness will soon disappear.

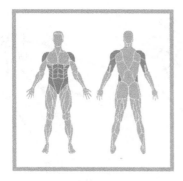

 up to you

Tai Chi

DAREBEE WORKOUT © darebee.com

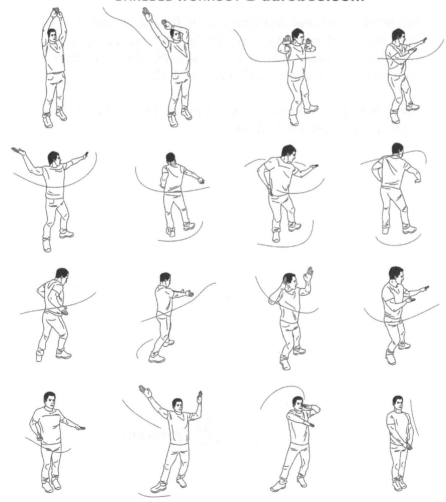

70 | The Walk

While taking a break from work to go for a walk and clear your mind and rejuvenate your body may sound great it is not always feasible. This is why The Walk allows you to do that just a few steps away from your desk.

What to watch: Coordinate your arms and legs so that they work in sync with each other.

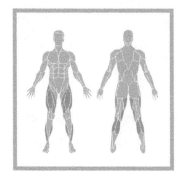

 2 minutes

the WALK

DAREBEE WORKOUT © darebee.com

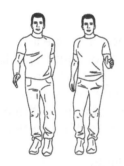

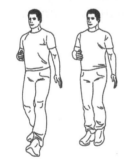

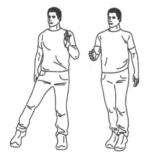

20sec walk on the spot

10sec heel to toe (left foot)

step to the right

20sec walk on the spot

10sec heel to toe (right foot)

step to the left

20sec walk on the spot

10sec heel to toe (left foot)

step to the right

20sec walk on the spot

10sec heel to toe (right foot)

step to the left

Done.

71 | Arms & Chest

Better flexibility helps improve your performance in physical activities or decrease your risk of injury by helping your joints move through their full range of motion and enabling your muscles to work most effectively. And you really need to invest such a small slice of time to it that it makes sense to make it part of your daily office routine.

What to watch: Move your trunk and limbs slowly, deliberately taking care to achieve the fullest range of motion possible.

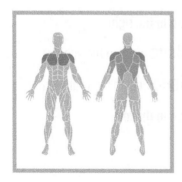

 2 minutes

arms & chest stretch

by DAREBEE
© darebee.com
20 seconds each exercise.

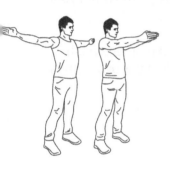

chest expansions

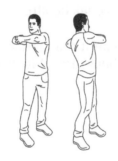

side-to-side torso twists

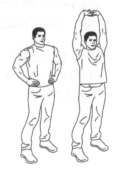

overhead stretch

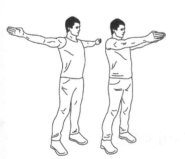

chest expansions

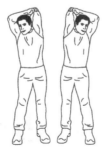

side-to-side tilts

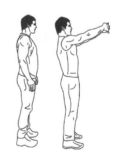

tricep stretches

72 | Arms & Shoulders

The shoulder is one of the most complicated joints in the body, it is actually two separate joints, combined. Our arms are used so much that they always take a pounding. A regular stretch routine that works both helps maintain your arms and shoulders in peak health.

What to watch: When performing tricep extensions push your arm all the way back, until it feels like your own arm is choking you.

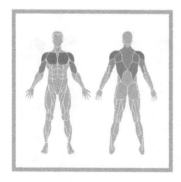

 2 minutes

arms
& shoulder
stretch

by DAREBEE
© **darebee.com**
20 seconds each exercise.

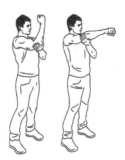

bicep extensions

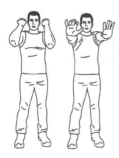

bicep extensions
both arms

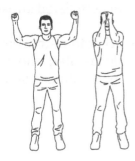

elbow clicks

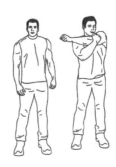

tricep expansions

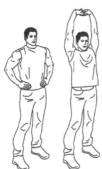

shoulder stretch

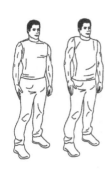

shoulder rotations

73 Back Pain Relief

Sitting down for most of the day takes its toll. Our back and shoulders are two areas specifically targeted by this workout that helps relieve aches and pains, ease muscle soreness and yes, even relieve some of the day's accumulated stress.

What to watch: Perform all trunk movements slowly, deliberately, allowing your body to slowly ease out of its joint stiffness and your spine to begin to move more freely.

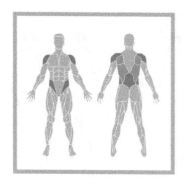

 2 minutes

stretching for back pain relief

by DAREBEE © darebee.com

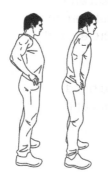
10 back and forth arches

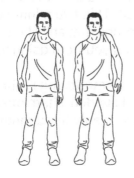
10 alternate shoulder raises

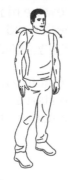
10 shoulder rotations

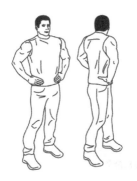
10 torso twists

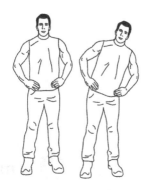
10 side-to-side bends

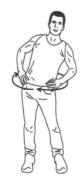
10 torso rotations

74 | Chest & Lower Back

Working the muscles and tendons of the chest and lower back can have a profound effect on how we feel and how we move and sit. This two minute workout can be performed any time, any day, anywhere so there are not many things stopping you from doing it.

What to watch: Like all stretching routines you need to start slowly, avoid sudden, sharp movements and remember to breathe evenly throughout.

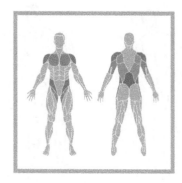

 2 minutes

chest & lower back stretch

by DAREBEE
© darebee.com
20 seconds each exercise.

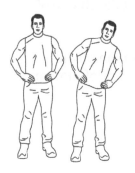

side bends

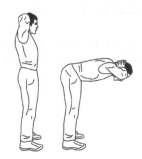

forward bends

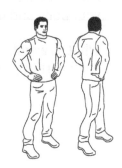

torso twists

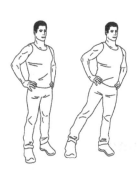

side leg raises

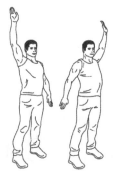

alt chest expansions

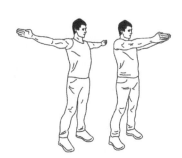

chest expansions

75 | Full Body Stretch

The number of productive days that are lost due to having unspecified aches and pains and a general feeling of discontent are almost immeasurable. The full body stretch workout counters that feeling. It helps you take charge of your body and feel great instantly.

What to watch: Go slow, move deliberately, manipulate each part of your body through its fullest range of motion.

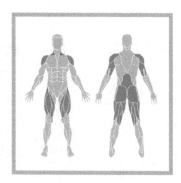

 4 minutes

full body stretch

by DAREBEE
© darebee.com
40 seconds
each exercise.

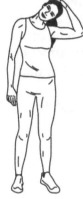

neck stretch

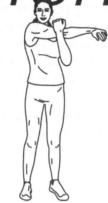

shoulder stretch

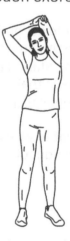

tricep stretch

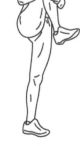

pelvic stretch

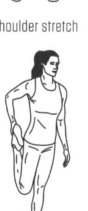

quad stretch

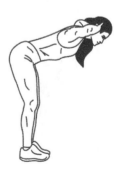

forward bend

76 | Glutes, Quads, Hamstrings & Calves

Our lower body doesn't only power us in practically everything we do it is also active while we are sat at our desk staring at a screen. A sore back, legs that ache or calves that feel like they have never worked hard affect our general disposition. This workout takes care of all of that.

What to watch: Keep your body as upright as possible throughout all of these exercises.

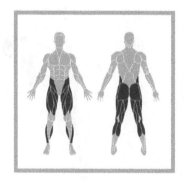

 2 minutes

Glutes, Quads, Hamstrings, & Calves

workout by DAREBEE
© darebee.com

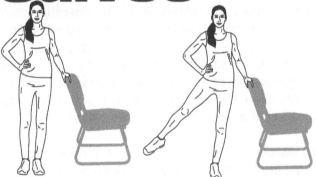

40 side leg raises

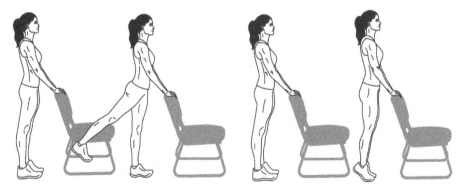

40 back kicks

40 calf raises

Reset Stretch

There is nothing more magical than being able to plug your body into a regeneration pod and after a few minutes feel like you have been completely reset. Regeneration pods are not a thing just yet, but the reset workout will help you stretch out the small knots of tension from your muscles, improve circulation and feel, in general, like you have been totally regenerated, plus it is totally eco-friendly as it uses none of the exotic energies a regeneration pod will require so you can do it anywhere, even at your desk.

What to watch: Like every stretching routine this too needs to be done slowly, deliberately with deep, even breathing to help you.

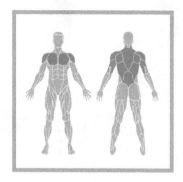

 2 minutes

Reset Stretch

DAREBEE WORKOUT © darebee.com
20 seconds each exercise.

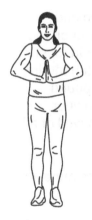

chest squeeze

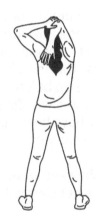

tricep stretch

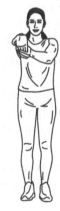

wrist stretch

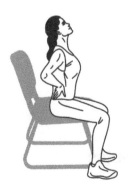

back arch

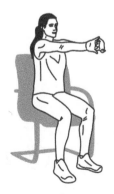

tricep stretch (both arms)

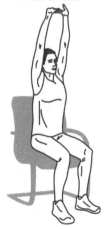

overhead shoulder stretch

78 | Shoulder Stretch

Because of typing, hunching in front of a screen and probably living through one Powerpoint presentation too many, shoulder tension is a common complaint in most offices and workplaces. This is a shoulder stretch routine that boxers use to limber up before starting to pound the heavy bag. It also works wonders at making your shoulders feel like they have been suddenly relieved of all the weight they've been carrying.

What to watch: Start slow and work the muscles more and more as your shoulders get warmed up.

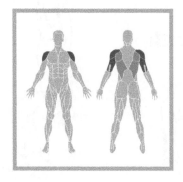

 2 minutes

shoulders
stretch

by DAREBEE © **darebee.com**
20 seconds each exercise.

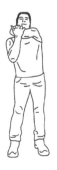

cross neck
stretch

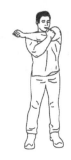

shoulder
stretch

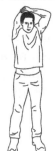

tricep
stretch

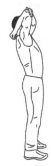

tricep
stretch #2

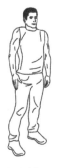

shoulders up
stretch

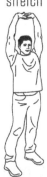

shoulder
& back stretch

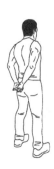

behind back
lock stretch

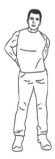

lock side pull
stretch

79 | Sitting Fix

Studies are constantly telling us how bad sitting all day is for us. For those of us who have no choice Sitting Fix is an easy way to undo all the potential damage sitting down does to us.

What to watch: You need to try and get as deep a stretch as possible here, but as always start slowly, listen to your body and try and work through the limitations you encounter in your range of motion.

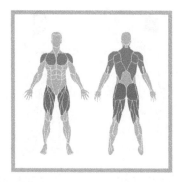

 2 minutes

sitting fix

DAREBEE WORKOUT © **darebee.com**
20 seconds each exercise.

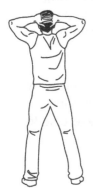

scapula stretch

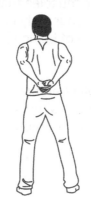

shoulder stretch

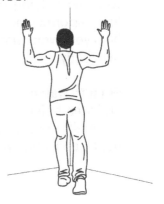

corner chest stretch

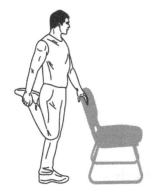

quad stretch

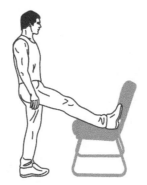

hamstring stretch

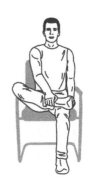

hip flexor stretch

80 | Upperbody Stretch

The upperbody stretch targets all of the trunk from the waist up, helping activate muscles that are tired by office life. Performed as part of your daily fitness routine it will help you avoid that feeling of being slow and heavy in your own body.

What to watch: As with all stretches you should start slow and steady, feeling your body's muscles work and then gradually increase the range of motion of each exercise to gently challenge you.

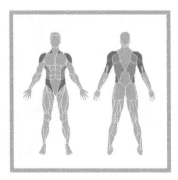

 2 minutes

upperbody
stretch

by DAREBEE © **darebee.com**
20 seconds each exercise.

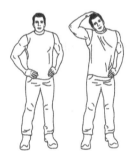

neck stretches

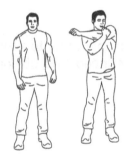

shoulder stretches

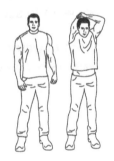

tricep stretches

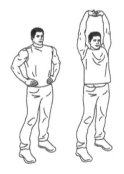

back & shoulders stretches

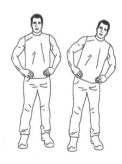

side bends

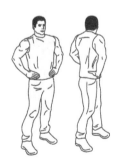

torso rotations

81 Arms 360

Despite the fact that we use our upperbody so much we generally have little proportional strength there. So every little we can do helps maintain upperbody health and strength and it accumulates towards the positive changes we want to see.

What to watch: Keep your arms to shoulder level on all exercises except the tricep dips, obviously.

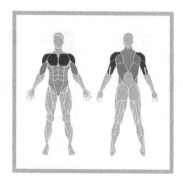

 15 minutes

arms 360

DAREBEE WORKOUT © **darebee.com**
repeat 3 times with 1 minute rest in between

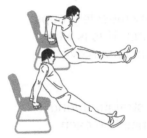

5 tricep dips

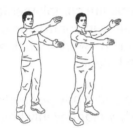

10 arm chops

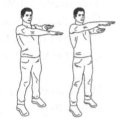

10 arm scissors

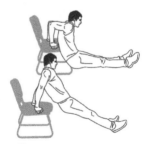

5 tricep dips

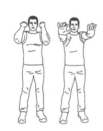

10 bicep extensions

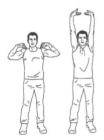

10 shoulder taps

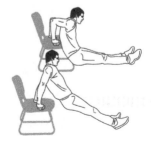

5 tricep dips

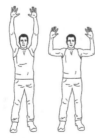

10 W-extensions

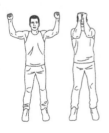

10 elbow clicks

82 | Biceps & Triceps

The biceps and triceps are complementary muscle groups. One supports and keeps in control the other. This is why working them both in one workout helps maintain overall upper body strength balance.

What to watch: Keep your body perfectly straight during these exercises, body weight evenly balanced on each foot.

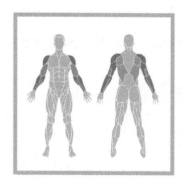

 15 minutes

biceps
& triceps LIGHT

DAREBEE WORKOUT © **darebee.com**
repeat 3 times with 1 minute rest in between

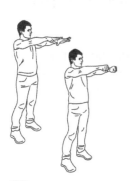

30 extended clench

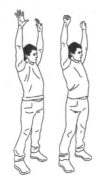

30 overhead clench

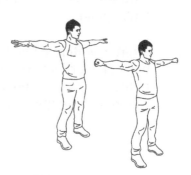

30 side extended clench

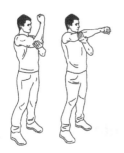

30 tricep extensions

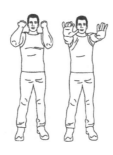

30 bicep extensions

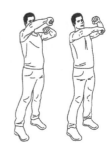

30 speed bag circles

83 | Boxer Arms

Boxers, of course, have phenomenal arm strength, speed and explosive power and they get it by practicing drills daily. Even small arm drills practiced regularly will go a long way towards helping you achieve great dexterity and limb speed.

What to watch: When throwing punches balance on the balls of your feet and swivel on the foot that is on the side of the arm you are punching with to transfer your body weight behind the punch, boxer style.

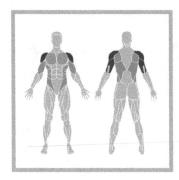

 15 minutes

Boxer Arms

DAREBEE WORKOUT © **darebee.com**
Repeat 3 times with 1 minute rest in between.
Keep arms up during the set.

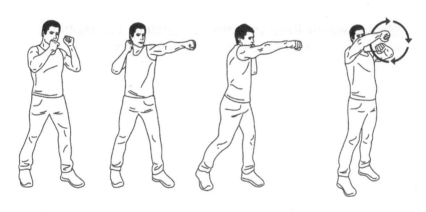

10 punches (jab + cross)

10 speed bag punches

20 punches (jab + cross)

20 speed bag punches

40 punches (jab + cross)

40 speed bag punches

done

84 | Chest & Back

Just because you work in an office doesn't mean you can't have toned chest and back muscles. The Chest & Back workout goes some way towards addressing this issue.

What to watch: Keep your arms as straight as possible in all exercises except the clasped arm rotations.

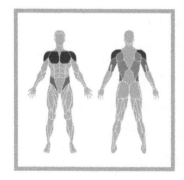

 15 minutes

chest & back
LIGHT

DAREBEE WORKOUT
© darebee.com
repeat 3 times
1 minute rest

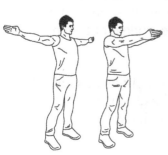

10 chest expansions

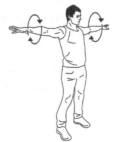

10 raised arm circles

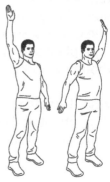

10 alt chest expansions

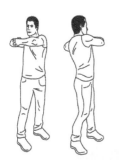

10 clasped arm rotations

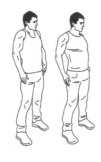

10 shoulder rotations

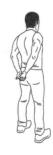

10-count shoulder stretch

85 | Chest & Shoulders

Using nothing but the weight of our own arms we can turn a few seemingly simple exercises into a satisfying upper body workout provided we use just the right angle. The Chest & Shoulders workout generates stress in all the right places to make you feel that you've worked out even though you never left the office.

What to watch: Maintain your arms as straight as possible throughout and bring them to shoulder height in all exercises bar the alternating chest expansions.

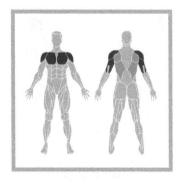

 15 minutes

chest & shoulders

DAREBEE WORKOUT © **darebee.com**
repeat 3 times with 1 minute rest in between

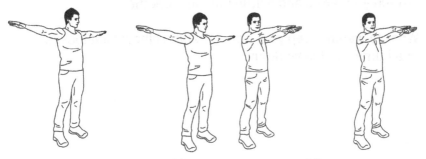

20sec raised arm hold   **20** chest expansions   **20sec** raised arm hold

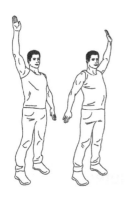   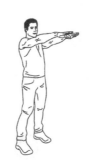   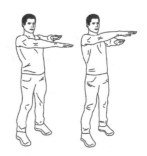

20 alt chest expansions   **20sec** raised arm hold   **20** arm scissors

86 | Forearms & Triceps

Forearms are necessary for a strong grip and tricep strength is required to power the arms' forward motion. Working either in the office requires just a little space to stretch your arms and a little time to work them.

What to watch: Keep your arms straight, elbow joint locked at all times in this workout.

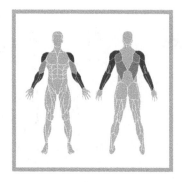

 15 minutes

forearms & triceps
LIGHT

DAREBEE WORKOUT © **darebee.com**
repeat 3 times with 1 minute rest in between

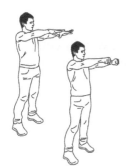

20 extended clench

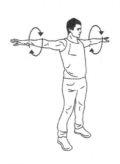

20 raised arm circles

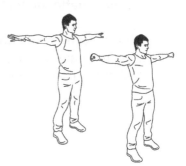

20 side extended clench

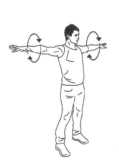

20 raised arm circles

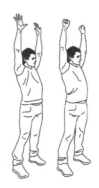

20 overhead clench

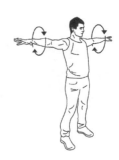

20 raised arm circles

87 | Office Push-Ups

Provided you have a wall that doesn't move you can transform it into a gym by using your body's weight to help provide the necessary resistance you need to develop and maintain better upper body strength.

What to watch: Just how much of your body's weight you bring to bear on your arms depends on the angle your body is at in relation to the wall.

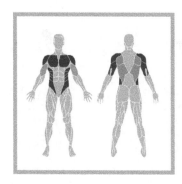

 10 minutes

Office Push-Ups

DAREBEE WORKOUT © darebee.com

88

Repeat 3 times with 1 minute rest in between.

10 wall push-ups

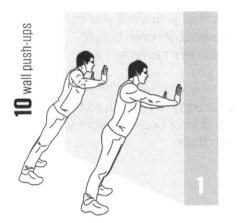

1

10 one-arm wall push-ups

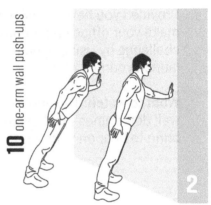

2

10 wall shoulder taps

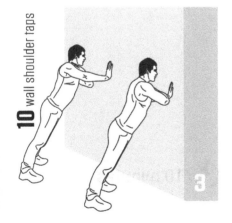

3

10 one-arm side wall push-ups

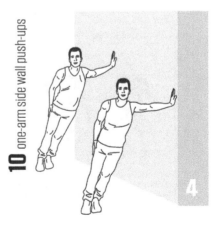

4

88 | Office Push-Ups II

Provided you have a wall handy, near your desk you can make your office upper body workout an even bigger challenge by using dynamic, explosive movements to launch yourself off it.

What to watch: The angle of your body in relation to the wall determines just how much of your body's weight you bring to bear on your arms, each time.

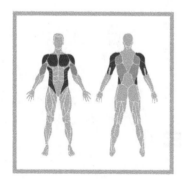

 10 minutes

Office Push-Ups II

DAREBEE WORKOUT © darebee.com

Repeat 3 times with 1 minute rest in between.

20 wall push-ups

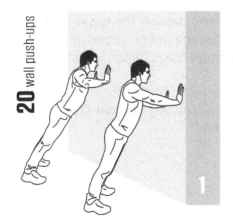

1

20 one-arm side wall push-ups

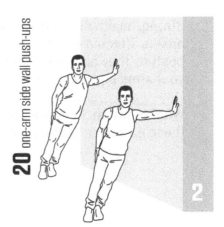

2

10 wall clapping push-ups

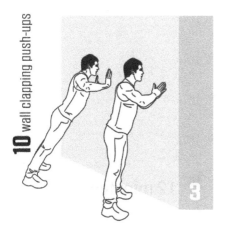

3

10 wall clapping push-ups behind back

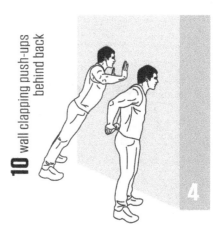

4

89 | Shoulder Work

Strong, healthy shoulders influence the way the lower neck area is affected which means they impact on your overall posture, they also help you do more basic things like lift your arms and carry things.

What to watch: Keep your arms absolutely straight during these exercises, elbow joint locked.

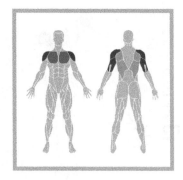

 12 minutes

shoulder work

DAREBEE WORKOUT
© **darebee.com**
repeat 3 times | 1 minute rest

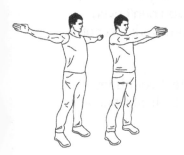

20 chest expansions

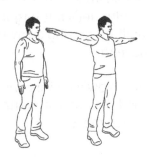

20 side arm raises

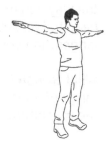

20sec raised arm hold

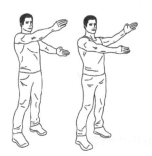

20 arm chops

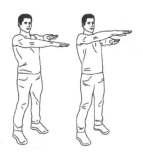

20 arm scissors

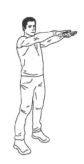

20sec raised arm hold

90 Upperbody Mobility

Shoulder mobility doesn't just require good joint flexibility, it also relies on unlocking the range of motion of the muscles on the neck and upper back region. This is what makes this workout so important to the way you feel and the way you move. Plus, let's not forget, you don't even need to feel any guilt for getting away from work a second longer than you have to.

What to watch: Start slowly on this one, test your body's range of motion and then as you warm up slowly increase the magnitude of each move.

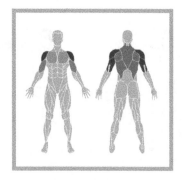

 12 minutes

upperbody
mobility

DAREBEE WORKOUT
© **darebee.com**
repeat 3 times
1 minute rest

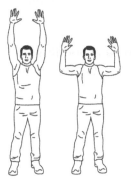

20 W-extensions

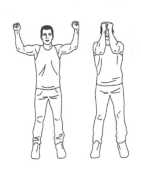

20 elbow clicks

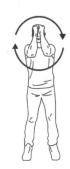

20 elbows together rotations

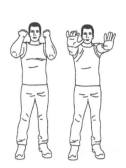

20 bicep extensions

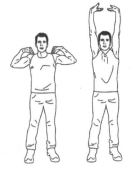

20 shoulder taps

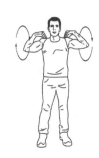

20 elbow rotations

91 | Back Fix

Transform your office chair into your Yoga buddy with this workout designed to help you stretch and stabilize all those important back muscles.

What to watch: No sudden movements. Go easy and flow into everything, watch how you breathe as you do so.

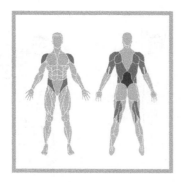

 2min 40 sec

back fix

DAREBEE WORKOUT © **darebee.com**

Hold each pose for 20 seconds.

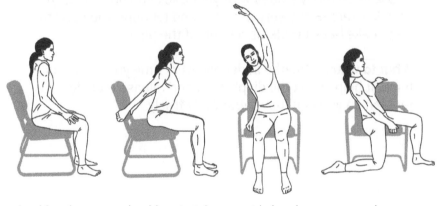

shoulder shrug	shoulder stretch	side bend	sea horse

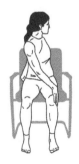 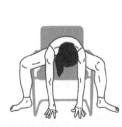 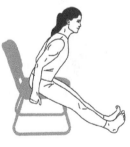 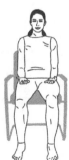

seated twist	wide leg fold	hamstring stretch	fall back

92 | Back Pain Relief (Chair)

It is only fitting that the chair you sit on which may be the cause of so many issues with your back can now be used to help exercise the very muscles and tendons you need to help make back problems a thing of the past.

What to watch: Breathe in deeply every time you arch your back. It helps relax the diaphragm and release muscle tension so you can move your body freely.

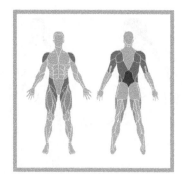

 2 minutes

BACK PAIN relief

chair edition

DAREBEE WORKOUT © darebee.com
Hold each pose for 20 seconds.

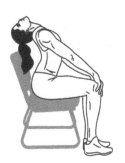

cat pose

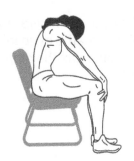

cow pose

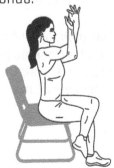

seated eagle pose

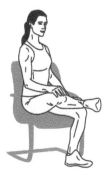

figure 4

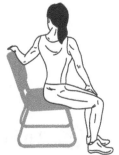

seated twist

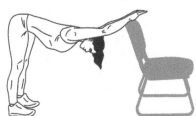

forward bend

93 | Back Pain Relief

With just a little space and a couple of minutes to burn you can use some exercises to completely transform the way your body moves and feels. You could then get back into the office swing of things feeling completely rejuvenated.

What to watch: Move slowly and deliberately. Assume as correct a pose as possible. Breathe in deeply every time you stretch your body to help relax the diaphragm muscles, exhale every time you fold it.

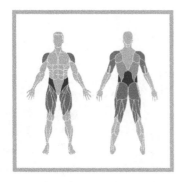

 2 minutes

BACK PAIN*relief*

YOGA WORKOUT
© **darebee.com**
Hold each pose
for 20 seconds.

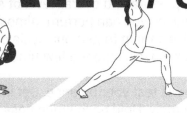
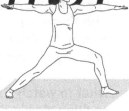

| forward bend | warrior I | warrior II |

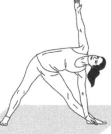
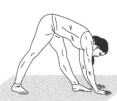
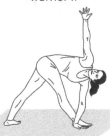

| triangle | side stretch | revolving triangle |

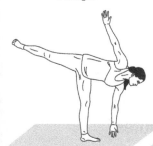
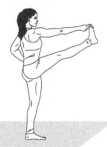

| half moon | warrior III | extended big toe hold |

94 | Balance

Improve your balance, posture and overall level of stability with these handy exercises you can perform almost anywhere. You could keep them to just one cycle or, as with any of the other exercises, repeat a few times.

What to watch: These will test your balance. Get into position slowly, deliberately. Hold each static pose for a full thirty seconds.

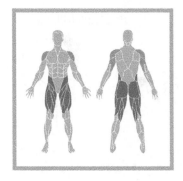

 3 minutes

balance *yoga*

DAREBEE WORKOUT
© darebee.com

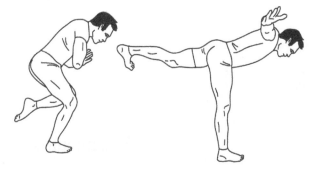

30seconds tree pose with reach, advance to - tree pose with reach, half squat

30seconds side leg raise, advance to - forward lg raise hold

30seconds single leg balance, advance to - warrior III pose

95 | Office Warrior

Warrior poses don't just look majestic, they also recruit all those muscle groups that, traditionally, a warrior in combat would have to call upon. Ok, you may not have to joust in the office or fight hordes of Orcs but that doesn't mean you can't exercise the same muscles to maintain your edge.

What to watch: Like all yoga exercises this too needs to be done deliberately and with care in your breathing. Allow your body to warm up into it without forcing it into positions until it is ready to flow into them.

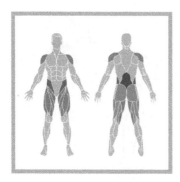

 2 minutes

office
WARRIOR

DAREBEE WORKOUT © **darebee.com**
Hold each pose for 20 seconds.

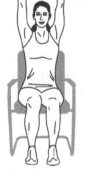

raised arms pose

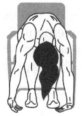

forward bend

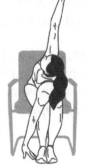

extended side angle

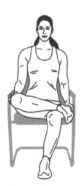

chair pigeon

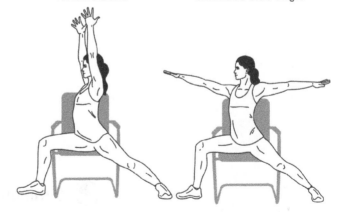

chair warrior I

chair warrior II

96 | Office Yoga

Turn your office chair into your Yoga buddy and feel the benefits of activating your body's primary muscle groups with a workout that's designed to make you feel like you've just come back from a spa.

What to watch: Move slowly, try and get into the entire range of motion of each movement. Exhale each time you lean forward and inhale deeply each time you stretch your body upwards to help relax the diaphragm.

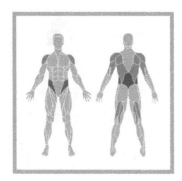

 2 minutes

office yoga

DAREBEE WORKOUT
© darebee.com
Hold each pose
for 20 seconds

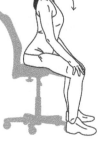

cat stretch

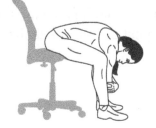

lower back stretch

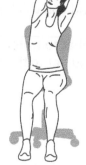

crescent pose

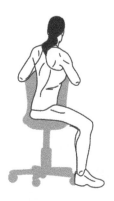

chair twist

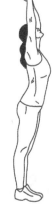

upward salute

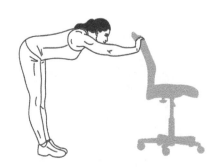

forward bend

97 | Origami

Time to test your flexibility and activate all those muscle groups and tendons that a hectic day at the office tends to put to sleep. You don't need to be super-flexible to try this and you will benefit regardless.

What to watch: Start counting the time from the moment you get to the deepest position of each pose.

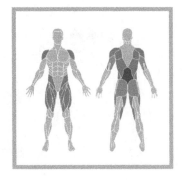

 2 minutes

origami
yoga

DAREBEE WORKOUT
© **darebee.com**
Hold each pose
for 20 seconds.

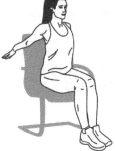

chest expansion

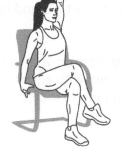

knee-over-knee reach

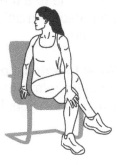

seated torso twist

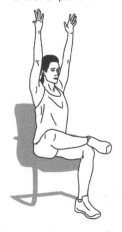

foot over knee reach

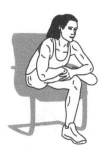

foot over knee fold

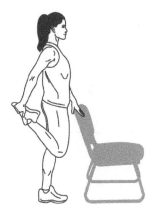

quad stretch

98 | Sun Salutation

There are few workouts you could do at work that will take you so completely out of your office reality and transport your mind to a time in the past when hardened warriors prepared themselves to greet a brand new day. This is one of them.

What to watch: Concentrate on your breathing. Feel your muscles relax and expand with each movement and synchronize your breathing to match.

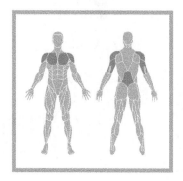

 2min 10 sec

Sun Salutation
chair edition

DAREBEE WORKOUT © **darebee.com**
Hold each pose for 10 seconds and move to the next one.

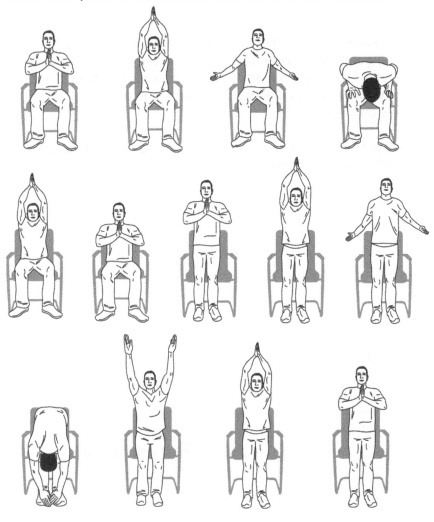

99 | Twist & Hold

Be brave. Be bold. Twist & Hold is a workout that will transform the way you feel about yourself and your body in very little time. But more than that, it will transform the way your mind connects to your body and revitalize you on any given day.

What to watch: Be aware of how your body moves as you perform each exercise.

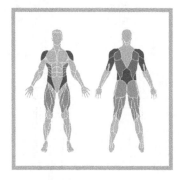

 2 min 40 sec

twist & fold

DAREBEE WORKOUT © darebee.com

Hold each move for 20 seconds.

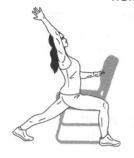

crescent lunge

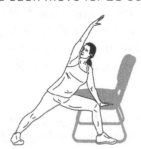

extended side angle

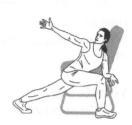

revolved side angle

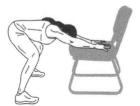

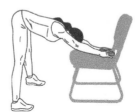

bent downward-facing dog - into - downward-facing dog

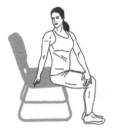

seated twist

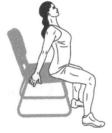

camel pose

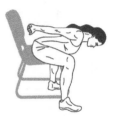

forward fold

100 Flow

On those days at the office when you feel you need to get a sense of flow back in your life this the workout that will give you what you crave, quickly and without having to roll out Yoga mats. You don't even have to leave your office chair.

What to watch: Exhale slowly as you bring your body together and inhale each time you begin to stretch.

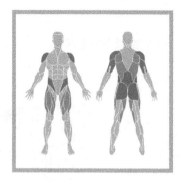

 2 minutes

yoga flow

DAREBEE WORKOUT
© **darebee.com**

Hold each pose
for 20 seconds.

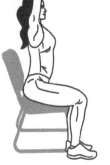

reach

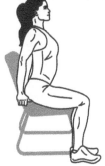

shoulders back

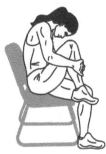

knee bend to cobra

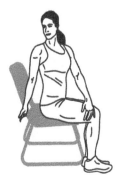

twist

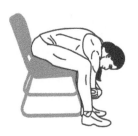

forward bend

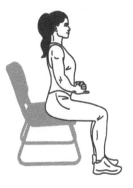

straight back

Thank you!

Thank you for purchasing *100 Office Workouts*, DAREBEE project print edition. DAREBEE is a non-profit global fitness resource dedicated to making fitness accessible for everyone, no matter their circumstances. The project is supported exclusively via user donations and paperback royalties.

After printing costs and store fees every book developed by the DAREBEE project makes $1 and it goes directly into our project maintenance and development fund.

Each sale helps us keep the DAREBEE resource growing, maintain it and keep it up. Thank you for making a difference in its future!